The Use of Drugs in the Care of the Sick

Ellen G. White

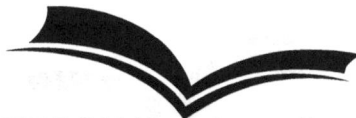

TEACH Services, Inc.
P U B L I S H I N G
www.TEACHServices.com • (800) 367-1844

Copyright © 2018 Ellen G. White
Copyright © 2018 TEACH Services, Inc.
ISBN-13: 978-1-4796-0913-0 (Paperback)
ISBN-13: 978-1-4796-0970-3 (ePub)
Library of Congress Control Number: 2018936249

The Use of Drugs in the Care of the Sick

A Compilation From the Writings of Ellen G. White

"After seeing so much harm done by the administering of drugs, I cannot use them, and cannot testify in the favor. I must be true to the light given me by the Lord" Letter 82 (1897).

Original Manuscript Compiled by Ellen G. White Publications
General Conference of S. D. A.
Washington, D. C.
March 18, 1954.

Additional statements on this topic may be found in Section 7 of *Selected Messages*, Book 2 (pp. 276–308).

Reprinted with the permission of the E.G. White Estate

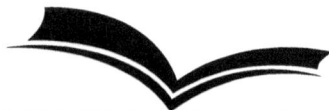

TEACH Services, Inc.
P U B L I S H I N G
www.TEACHServices.com • (800) 367-1844

Table of Contents

CHAPTER 1

Drugs and Their Use

(First E.G. White Statement, 1864)

(This first E.G. White presentation on Drugs was published in 1864 as a part of her initial 40-page article "Health," presenting the Health Reform Program.)

The Vision of June 6, 1863. I was shown that more deaths have been caused by drug-taking than from all other causes combined. If there was in the land one physician in the place of thousands, a vast amount of premature mortality would be prevented. Multitudes of physicians, and multitudes of drugs, have cursed the inhabitants of the earth, and have carried thousands and tens of thousands to untimely graves.

Indulging in eating too frequently, and in too large quantities, overtaxes the digestive organs, and produces a feverish state of the system. The blood becomes impure, and then diseases of various kinds occur. A physician is sent for, who prescribes some drug which gives present relief, but which does not cure the disease. It may change the form of disease, but the real evil is increased ten fold. Nature was doing her best to rid the system of an accumulation of impurities, and could she have been left to herself, aided by the common blessings of heaven, such as pure air and pure water, a speedy and safe cure would have been affected.

The sufferers in such cases can do for themselves that which others cannot do as well for them. They should commence to relieve nature of the load they have forced upon her. They should remove the cause, fast a short time, and give the stomach chance for rest. Reduce the feverish state of the system by a careful and understanding application of water. These efforts will help nature in her struggles to free the system of impurities. But generally the persons who suffer pain become impatient. They are not willing to use self-denial, and suffer a little from hunger. Neither are they willing to wait for the slow process of nature to build up the overtaxed energies of the system. But they are determined to obtain relief at once, and take powerful drugs, prescribed by physicians. Nature was doing her work well, and would have triumphed, but while accomplishing her task, a foreign substance of a poisonous nature was introduced. What a mistake! Abused nature has now two evils to war against instead of one. She leaves the work in which she was engaged, and resolutely takes hold to expel the intruder newly introduced into the system. Nature feels this double draft upon her resources, and she becomes enfeebled.

Drugs never cure disease. They only change the form and location. Nature alone is the effectual restorer, and how much better could she perform her task if left to herself. But this privilege is seldom allowed her. If crippled nature bears up under the load, and finally accomplishes in a great measure her double task, and the patient lives, the credit is given to the physician. But if nature fails in her effort to expel the poison from the system, and the patient dies, it is called a wonderful dispensation of Providence. If the patient had taken a course to relieve over burdened nature in season, and understandingly used pure soft water, this dispensation of drug mortality might have been wholly averted. The use of water can accomplish but little, if the patient does not feel the necessity of also strictly attending to his diet.

Many are living in violation of the laws of health, and are ignorant of the relation their habits of eating, drinking, and working sustain to their health. They will not arouse to their true condition until nature protests against the abuses she is suffering, by aches and pains in the system. If, even then, the sufferers would only commence the work right, and would resort to the simple means they have neglected—the use of water and proper diet, nature would have just the help she requires, and which she ought to have had long before. If this course is pursued, the patient will generally recover, without being debilitated.

When drugs are introduced into the system, for a time they may seem to have a beneficial effect. A change may take place, but the disease is not cured. It will manifest itself in some other form. In nature's efforts to expel the drug from the system, intense suffering is sometimes caused the patient. And the disease, which the drug was given to cure, may disappear, but only to reappear in a new form, such as skin diseases, ulcers, painful diseased joints, and sometimes in a more dangerous and deadly form. The liver, heart and brain are frequently affected by drugs, and often all these organs are burdened with disease, and the unfortunate subjects, if they live, are invalids for life, wearily dragging out a miserable existence. Oh, how much that poisonous drug cost! If it did not cost the life, it cost quite too much. Nature has been crippled in all her efforts. The whole machinery is out of order, and at a future period in life, when these fine works which have been injured, are to be relied upon to act a more important part in union with all the fine works of nature's machinery, they cannot readily and strongly perform their labor, and the whole system feels the lack. These organs, which should be in a healthy condition, are enfeebled, the blood becomes impure. Nature keeps struggling, and the patient suffers with different ailments, until there is a sudden breaking down in her efforts, and death follows. There are more who die from the use of drugs, than all who would have died of disease had nature been left to do her own work.

Uncertainty in Diagnosis. Very many lives have been sacrificed by physicians' administering drugs for unknown diseases. They have no real knowledge of the exact disease which afflicts the patient. But physicians are expected to know in a moment what to do, and unless they act at once, as though they understood the disease perfectly, they are considered by impatient friends, and by the sick, as incompetent physicians. Therefore to gratify erroneous opinions of the sick and their friends, medicine must be administered, experiments and tests tried to cure the patient of the disease of which they have no real knowledge. Nature is loaded with poisonous drugs which she cannot expel from the system. The physicians themselves are often convinced that they have used powerful medicines for a disease which did not exist, and death was the consequence.

Physicians are censurable, but they are not the only ones at fault. The sick themselves, if they would be patient, diet and suffer a little, and give nature time to rally, would recover much sooner without the use of any medicine. NATURE ALONE POSSESSES CURATIVE POWERS. Medicines have no power to cure, but will most generally hinder nature in her efforts. She after all must do the work of restoring. The sick are in a hurry to get well, and the friends of the sick are impatient. They will have medicine, and if they do not feel that powerful influence upon their systems, their erroneous views lead them to think they should feel, they impatiently change for another physician. The change often increases the evil. They go through a course of medicine equally as dangerous as the first, and more fatal, because the two treatments do not agree, and the system is poisoned beyond remedy.

The Use of Water for Fever Cases. But many have never experienced the beneficial effects of water, and are afraid to use one of heaven's greatest blessings. Water has been refused persons suffering with burning fevers, through fear that it would injure them. If, in their fevered state, water had been given them to drink freely, and applications had also been made externally, long days and nights of suffering would have been saved, and many precious lives spared. But thousands have died with raging fevers consuming them, until the fuel which fed the fever was burnt up, the vitals consumed, and have died in the greatest agony, without being permitted to have water to allay their burning thirst. Water, which is allowed a senseless building, to put out the raging elements, is not allowed human beings to put out the fire which is consuming the vitals.

Inexcusable Ignorance. Multitudes remain in inexcusable ignorance in regard to the laws of their being. They are wondering why our race is so feeble, and why so many die prematurely. Is there not a cause? Physicians who profess to understand the human organism, prescribe for their patients, and even for their own dear children, and their companions, slow poisons to break up disease, or to cure slight indisposition. Surely, they cannot realize the evil of these things as they were presented before me, or they could not do thus. The effects of the poison may not be immediately perceived, but it is doing its work surely in the system, undermining the constitution, and crippling nature in her efforts. They are seeking to correct an evil, but produce a far greater one, which is often incurable.

Drug Invalidism. Those who are thus dealt with are constantly sick, and constantly dosing. And yet, if you listen to their conversation, you will often hear them praising the drugs they have been using, and recommending their use to others, because they have been benefited by their use. It would seem that to such as can reason from cause to effect, the sallow countenance, the continual complaints of ailments and general prostration of those who claim to be benefited, would be sufficient proofs of the health-destroying influence of drugs. And yet many are so blinded they do not see that all the drugs they have taken have not cured them, but made them worse. The drug invalid numbers one in the world, but is generally peevish, irritable, always sick, lingering out a miserable existence, and seems to live only to call into constant exercise the patience of others. Poisonous drugs have not killed them outright, for nature is loth to give up her hold on life. She is unwilling to cease her struggles. Yet these drug-takers are never well. They are always taking cold, which causes extreme suffering, because of the poison all through their system.

Strychnine. A branch was presented before me bearing large flat seeds. Upon it was written, NUX VOMICA, STRYCHNINE. Beneath was written, NO ANTIDOTE. I was shown persons under the influence of this poison. It produced heat, and seemed to act particularly on the spinal column, but affected the whole system. When this is taken in the smallest quantities, it has its influence, which nothing can counteract. If taken immoderately, convulsions, paralysis, insanity, and death are often the results. Many use this deadly evil in small quantities. But if they realized its influence, not one grain of it would be introduced into the system.

When first taken, its influence may seem to be beneficial. It excites the nerves connected with the spinal column, but when the excitement passes away, it is followed by a sense of prostration and of chilliness the whole length of the spinal column, especially upon the head and back of the neck. The patients generally cannot endure the least draught of air. They are inclined to close every crevice, and for want of the free, invigorating air of heaven, the blood becomes impure, the vital organs are weakened, and general debility is the result. By unduly exciting the sensitive nerves connected with the spinal column, by this poisonous drug, they lose their tone and vitality, and weakness of the back and limbs follows. The sight and hearing are often affected, and in many cases the patient becomes helpless.

Opium. I was shown that the innocent, modest-looking, white poppy yields a dangerous drug. Opium is a slow poison, when taken in small quantities. In large doses it produces lethargy and death. Its effects upon the nervous system are ruinous. When patients use this drug until it becomes habit, it is almost impossible to discontinue it, because they feel so prostrated and nervous without it. They are in a worse condition when deprived of it than the rum-drinker without his rum, or the tobacco-user deprived of his tobacco. The opium slave is in a pitiful condition. Unless his nervous system is continually intoxicated with the poisonous drug, he is miserable. It benumbs the sensibilities, stupefies the brain, and unfits the mind for the service of God. True Christians cannot persist in the use of this slow poison, when they know its influence upon them.

Those who use opium cannot render to God any more acceptable service than can the drunkard, or the tobacco-user. Those who break off the use of this nerve-and-brain-destroying practice will have to possess fortitude, and suffer, as will the drunkard and the tobacco slave, when deprived of their body-and-mind-destroying indulgences. God is displeased that His followers should become slaves to habits which ruin body and mind. Nux vomica, or strychnine, and opium have killed their millions, and have left thousands upon the earth to linger out a wretched, suffering existence, a burden to themselves, and those around them.

Mercury, Calomel, Quinine. Mercury, calomel, and quinine have brought their amount of wretchedness, which the day of God alone will fully reveal. Preparations of mercury and calomel taken into the system ever retain their poisonous strength as long as there is a particle of it left in the system. Theses poisonous preparations have destroyed their millions, and left sufferers upon the earth to linger out a miserable existence. All are better off without these dangerous mixtures. Miserable sufferers, with disease in almost every form, misshapen by suffering, with dreadful ulcers, and pains in the bones, loss of teeth, loss of memory, and impaired sight, are to be seen almost everywhere. They are victims of poisonous preparations, which have been, in many cases, administered to cure some slight indisposition, which after a day or two of fasting would have disappeared without medicine. But poisonous mixtures, administered by physicians, have proved their ruin.

The Drug Evil. The endless variety of medicines in the market, the numerous advertisements of new drugs and mixtures, all of which, they say, do wonderful cures, kill hundreds where they benefit one. Those who are sick are not patient. They will take the various medicines, some of which are very powerful, although they know nothing of the nature of the mixtures. All the medicines they take only make their recovery more hopeless. Yet they keep dosing, and continue to grow weaker, until they die. Some will have medicine at all events. Then let them take these hurtful mixtures and the various deadly poisons upon their own responsibility. God's servants should not administer medicines which they know will leave behind injurious effects upon the system, even if they do relieve present suffering.

Every poisonous preparation in the vegetable and mineral kingdoms, taken into the system, will leave its wretched influence, affecting the liver and lungs, and deranging the system generally. Nor does the evil end here. Diseased, feeble infants are brought into the world to share this misery, transmitted to them from their parents.

Spiritual Gifts, Vol. IV, pp. 133–140.

CHAPTER 2

A Vivid Presentation of the Effects of Drugs

(Second E.G. White Statement, 1865)

(The second E.G. White statement on Drugs was published in 1865 in HOW TO LIVE, Number 3, in an article entitled "Disease and Its Causes.")

The Use of Powerful Poisons. The human family have brought upon themselves diseases of various forms by their own wrong habits. They have not studied how to live healthfully, and their transgression of the laws of their being has produced a deplorable state of things. The people have seldom accredited their sufferings to the true cause—their own wrong course of action. They have indulged in intemperance in eating, and made a god of their appetite. In all their habits they have manifested a recklessness in regard to health and life; and when, as the result, sickness has come upon them, they have made themselves believe that God was the author of it, when their own wrong course of action has brought the sure result. When in distress, they send for the doctor, and trust their bodies in his hands, expecting that he will make them well. He deals out to them drugs, of the nature of which they know nothing; and in their blind confidence they swallow anything that the doctor may choose to give. Thus powerful poisons are often administered, which fetter nature in all her friendly efforts to recover from the abuse the system has suffered; and the patient is hurried out of this life.

The mother who has been but slightly indisposed, and who might have recovered by abstaining from food for a short period, and ceasing from labor, having quiet and rest, has, instead of doing this, sent for a physician. And he, who should be prepared to give a few simple directions, and restrictions in diet, and place her upon the right track, is either too ignorant to do this, or too anxious to obtain a fee.

Some Drugged to Death. He makes the case appear a grave one, and administers his poisons, which, if he himself were sick, he would not venture to take. The patient grows worse, and poisonous drugs are more freely administered, until nature is overpowered in her efforts, and gives up the conflict, and the mother dies. She was drugged to death. Her system was poisoned beyond remedy. She was murdered. Neighbors and relatives marvel at the wonderful dealings of Providence in thus removing a mother in the midst of her usefulness, at the period when her children need her care so much. They wrong our good and wise Heavenly Father when they cast back upon Him this weight of human woe. Heaven wished that mother to live, and her untimely death dishonored God. The mother's wrong habits, and her inattention to the law of her being, made her sick. And the doctor's fashionable poisons, introduced into the system, closed the period of her existence, and left a helpless, stricken, motherless flock.

This is not always the result which follows the doctor's drugging. Sick people who take these drug-poisons do appear to get well. With some, there is sufficient life-force for nature to draw upon, to so far expel the poison from the system that the sick, having a period of rest, recover. But no credit should be allowed the drugs taken, for they only hindered nature in her efforts. ALL THE CREDIT SHOULD BE ASCRIBED TO NATURE'S RESTORATIVE POWERS.

Although the patient may recover, yet the powerful effort nature was required to make to induce action to overcome the poison, injured the constitution, and shortened the life of the patient. There are many who do not die under the influence of drugs; but there are very many who are left useless wrecks, hopeless, gloomy, and miserable sufferers, a burden to themselves and to society.

They Deteriorate the Race. If those who take these drugs were alone the sufferers, then the evil would not be so great. Parents not only sin against themselves in swallowing drug-poisons, but they sin against their children. The vitiated state of their blood, the poison distributed throughout the system, the broken constitution, and various drug-diseases, as the result of drug-poisons, are transmitted to their offspring, and left to them as a wretched inheritance. This is another great cause of the degeneracy of the race.

Physicians, by administering their drug-poisons, have done very much to increase the deterioration of the race, physically, mentally, and morally. Everywhere you may go you will see deformity, disease, and imbecility, which in very many cases can be traced directly back to the drug-poisons administered by the hand of a doctor as a remedy for some of life's ills. The so-called remedy has fearfully proved itself to the patient, by stern, suffering experience, to be far worse than the disease for which the drug was taken. All who possess common capabilities should understand the wants of their own systems. The philosophy of health should compose one of the important studies for our children. It is all-important that the human organism be understood; then intelligent men and women can be their own physicians. If the people would reason from cause to effect, and would follow the light which shines upon them, they would pursue a course which would insure health, and mortality would be far less. But the people are too willing to remain in inexcusable ignorance, and trust their bodies to the doctors, instead of having any special responsibility themselves.

Four Illustrative Cases. Several illustrations of this great subject have been presented before me. The first was a family consisting of a father and daughter. The daughter was sick, and the father was much troubled on her account, and summoned a physician. As the father conducted him into the sick-room, he manifested a painful anxiety. The physician examined the patient, and said but little. They both left the sick-room. The father informed the physician that he had buried the mother, a son, and a daughter, and that this daughter was all that was left to him of his family. He anxiously inquired of the physician if he thought his daughter's case hopeless.

The physician then inquired in regard to the nature and length of the sickness of those who had died. The father mournfully related the painful facts connected with the illness of his loved ones. "My son was first attacked with a fever. I called a physician. He said that he could administer medicine which would soon break the fever. He gave him powerful medicine, but was disappointed in its effects. The fever was reduced, but my son grew dangerously sick. The same medicine was again given him, without producing any change for the better. The physician then resorted to still more powerful medicines, but my son obtained no relief. The fever left him, but he did not rally. He sank rapidly and died.

"The death of my son, so sudden and unexpected, was a great grief to us all, especially to his mother. Her watching and anxiety in his sickness, and her grief, occasioned by his sudden death, were too much for her nervous system, and she was soon prostrated. I felt dissatisfied with the course pursued by this physician. My confidence in his skill was shaken, and I could not employ him a second time. I called another to my suffering wife. This second physician gave her a liberal dose of opium, which he said would relieve her pain, quiet her nerves, and give her rest, which she much needed. The opium stupefied her. She slept, and nothing could arouse her from the deathlike stupor. Her pulse and heart at times throbbed violently, and then grew more and more feeble in their action, until she ceased to breathe. Thus she died, without giving her family one look of recognition. This second death seemed more than we could endure. We all sorrowed deeply; but I was agonized, and could not be comforted.

"My daughter was next afflicted. Grief, anxiety, and watching had overtasked her powers of endurance, and her strength gave way, and she was brought upon a bed of suffering. I had now lost confidence in both of the physicians I had employed. Another physician was recommended to me as being successful in treating the sick; and although he lived at a distance, I was determined to obtain his services.

"This third physician professed to understand my daughter's case. He said that she was greatly debilitated, that her nervous system was deranged, and that fever was upon her, which could be controlled, but that it would take time to bring her up from her present state of debility. He expressed perfect confidence in his ability to raise her. He gave her powerful medicine to break up the fever. This was accomplished. But as the fever left, the case assumed more alarming features, and grew more complicated. As the symptoms changed, the medicines were varied to meet the case. While under the influence of new medicines, she would, for a time, appear revived. This would flatter our hopes that she would get well, only to make our disappointment more bitter as she became worse.

"The physician's last resort was calomel. For some time she seemed to be between life and death. She was thrown into convulsions. As these most distressing spasms ceased, we were aroused to the painful fact that her intellect was weakened. She began slowly to improve, although still a great sufferer. Her limbs were crippled as the effect of the powerful poisons which she had taken. She lingered a few years, a helpless, pitiful sufferer, and died in much agony."

After this sad relation the father looked imploringly to the physician, and entreated him to save his only remaining child. The physician looked sad and anxious, but made no prescription. He arose to leave, saying that he would call the next day.

Three Cases Treated With Drugs. Another scene was then presented before me. I was brought into the presence of a female, apparently about thirty years of age. A physician was standing by her, and reporting that her nervous system was deranged, that her blood was impure and moved sluggishly, and that her stomach was in a cold, inactive condition. He said he would give her active remedies, which would soon improve her condition. He gave her a powder from a vial upon which was written "Nux vomica." I watched to see what effect this would have upon the patient. It appeared to act favorably. Her condition seemed better. She was animated, and even seemed cheerful and active.

My attention was then called to still another case. I was introduced into the sick-room of a young man who was in a high fever. A physician was standing by the bedside of the sufferer, with a portion of medicine taken from a vial upon which was written "Calomel." He administered this chemical poison, and a change seemed to take place, but not for the better.

I was then shown still another case. It was that of a female, who seemed to be suffering much pain. A physician stood by the bedside of the patient, and was administering medicine taken from a vial upon which was written "Opium." At first this drug seemed to affect the mind. She talked strangely, but finally became quiet, and slept.

Back to the Anxious Father. My attention was then called to the first case, that of the father who had lost his wife and two children. The physician was in the sick-room, standing by the bedside of the afflicted daughter. Again he left the room without giving medicine. The father, when alone in the presence of the physician, seemed deeply moved, and inquired, impatiently, "Do you intend to do nothing? Will you leave my only daughter to die?"

The physician said: "I have listened to the sad history of the death of your much-loved wife and your two children, and have learned from your own lips that all three died while in the care of physicians, and while taking medicines prescribed and administered by their hands. Medicine has not saved your loved ones; and as a physician, I solemnly believe that none of them need, or ought to, have died. They could have recovered if they had not been so drugged that nature was enfeebled by abuse, and finally crushed." He stated decidedly to the agitated father: "I cannot give medicine to your daughter. I shall only seek to assist nature in her efforts, by removing every obstruction, and then leave nature to recover the exhausted energies of the system." He placed in the father's hand a few directions, which he enjoined him to follow closely: "Keep the patient free from excitement, and every influence calculated to depress. Her attendants should be cheerful and hopeful. She should have a simple diet, and should be allowed plenty of pure soft water to drink. She should bathe frequently in pure soft water, and this treatment should be followed by gentle rubbing. Let light and air be freely admitted into her room. She must have quiet and undisturbed rest."

The father slowly read the prescription, wondered at the few simple directions it contained, and seemed doubtful that any good would result from such simple means.

Said the physician: "You have had sufficient confidence in my skill to place the life of your daughter in my hands. Withdraw not your confidence. I will visit your daughter daily, and direct you in the management of her case. Follow my directions with confidence, and I trust in a few weeks to present her to you in a much better condition of health, if not fully restored."

The father looked sad and doubtful, but submitted to the decision of the physician. He feared that his daughter must die, if she had no medicine.

Program of the Other Cases. The second case was again presented before me. The patient had appeared better under the influence of nux vomica. She was sitting up, folding a shawl closely around her, and complaining of chilliness. The air in the room was impure. It was heated, and had lost its vitality. Almost every crevice where pure air could enter was guarded, to protect the patient from a sense of painful chilliness, which was especially felt in the back of the neck and down the spinal column. If the door was left ajar, she seemed nervous and distressed, and entreated that it should be closed, for she was cold. She could not bear the least draft of air from the door or windows. A gentleman of intelligence stood looking pityingly upon her, and said, to those present: "This is the second result of nux vomica. It is especially felt upon the nerves, and it affects the whole nervous system. There will be, for a time, increased forced action upon the nerves. But as the strength of this drug is spent, there will be chilliness and prostration. Just to the degree that it excites and enlivens will be the deadening, benumbing results following."

The third case was again presented before me. It was that of the young man to whom was administered calomel. He was a great sufferer. His lips were dark and swollen. His gums were inflamed. His tongue was thick and swollen, and the saliva was running from his mouth in large quantities. The intelligent gentleman before mentioned looked sadly upon the sufferer, and said: "This is the influence of mercurial preparations. This young man had sufficient nervous energy remaining to begin a warfare upon this intruder, this drug poison, to attempt to expel it from the system. Many have not sufficient life-force left to arouse to action; and nature is overpowered, ceases her efforts, and the victim dies."

The fourth case, the person to whom was given opium, was again presented before me. She had awakened from her sleep much prostrated. Her mind was distracted. She was impatient and irritable, finding fault with her best friends, and imagining that they did not try to relieve her sufferings. She became frantic, and raved like a maniac. The gentleman before mentioned looked sadly upon the sufferer, and said to those present: "This is the second result of taking opium."

Her physician was called. He gave her an increased dose of opium, which quieted her ravings, yet made her very talkative and cheerful. She was at peace with all around her, and expressed much affection for acquaintances, as well as for her relatives. She soon grew drowsy, and fell into a stupefied condition. The gentleman mentioned above, solemnly said: "Her condition is no better now than when she was in her frantic ravings. She is decidedly worse. This drug-poison, opium, gives temporary relief from pain, but does not remove the cause of pain. It only stupefies the brain, rendering it incapable of receiving impressions from the nerves. While the brain is thus insensible, the hearing, the taste, and the sight are affected. When the influence of opium wears off, and the brain arouses from its state of paralysis, the nerves, which had been cut off from communication with the brain, shriek out, louder than ever, the pain in the system, because of the additional outrage the system has sustained in receiving this poison. Every additional drug given to the patient, whether it be opium or some other poison, will complicate the case, and make the patient's recovery more hopeless. The drugs given to stupefy, whatever they may be, derange the nervous system. An evil, simple in the beginning, which nature aroused herself to overcome, and which she would have overcome had she been left to herself, has been made tenfold worse by the introduction of drug-poisons into the system. The result of these poisons is a destructive disease of itself, forcing into extraordinary action the remaining life forces to war against and overcome the drug intruder."

Gratifying Results in the First Case. I was brought again into the sick-room of the first case, that of the father and his daughter. The daughter was sitting by the side of her father, cheerful and happy, with the glow of health upon her countenance. The father was looking upon her with happy satisfaction, his countenance speaking the gratitude of his heart, that his only child was spared to him. Her physician entered, and after conversing with the father and child for a short time, arose to leave. He addressed the father thus: "I present to you your daughter restored to health. I gave her no medicine, that I might leave her with an unbroken constitution. Medicine never could have accomplished this. Medicine deranges nature's fine machinery, and breaks down the constitution, and kills, but it never cures. NATURE ALONE POSSESSES RESTORATIVE POWERS. She alone can build up her exhausted energies, and repair the injuries she has received by inattention to her fixed laws."

He then asked the father if he was satisfied with his manner of treatment. The happy father expressed his heartfelt gratitude and perfect satisfaction, saying: "I have learned a lesson I shall never forget. It was painful, yet it is of priceless value. I am now convinced that my wife and children need not have died. Their lives were sacrificed while in the hands of physicians, by their poisonous drugs."

Results of Drugging. I was then shown the second case—the patient to whom nux vomica had been administered. She was being supported by two attendants, from her chair to her bed. She had nearly lost the use of her limbs. The spinal nerves were partially paralyzed, and the limbs had lost their power to bear her weight. She coughed distressingly, and breathed with difficulty. She was laid upon the bed, and soon lost her hearing and sight; and after lingering thus a while, she died. The gentleman before mentioned looked sorrowfully upon the lifeless body, and said to those present: "Witness the protracted influence of nux vomica upon the human system. At its introduction, the nervous energy was excited to extraordinary action to meet this drug-poison. This extra excitement was followed by prostration, and the final result has been paralysis of the nerves. This drug does not have the same effect upon all. Some, who have powerful constitutions; recover from abuses to which they may subject the system; while others, whose hold on life is not so strong, who possess enfeebled constitutions, never recover from receiving into the system even one dose; many die from no other cause than the effects of one portion of this poison. Its effects are always tending to death. The condition the system is in, at the time those poisons are received into it, determines the life of the patient. Nux vomica can cripple, paralyze, destroy health forever, but it never cures."

The third case—that of the young man to whom had been administered calomel—was again presented before me. He was a pitiful sufferer. His limbs were crippled, and he was greatly deformed. He said that his sufferings were beyond description, and life was to him a great burden. The gentleman whom I have repeatedly mentioned looked upon the sufferer with sadness and pity, and said: "This is the effect of calomel. It torments the system as long as there is a particle of the poison left in it. It ever lives, not losing its properties by its long stay in the living system. It inflames the joints, and often sends rottenness into the bones. It frequently manifests itself in the tumors, ulcers, and cancers, years after it has been introduced into the system."

The fourth case was again presented before me —the patient to whom opium had been administered. Her countenance was sallow, and her eyes were restless and glassy. Her hands shook as if palsied, and she appeared greatly excited, imagining that all present were leagued against her. Her mind was a complete wreck, and she raved in a pitiful manner. The physician was summoned, and seemed to be unmoved at these terrible exhibitions. He gave the patient a more powerful portion of opium, which he said would set her all right. Her ravings did not cease until she became thoroughly intoxicated. She then passed into a deathlike stupor. The gentleman already mentioned looked upon the patient, and said, sadly: "Her days are numbered. The efforts that nature has made have been so many times overpowered by this poison that the vital forces are exhausted by being repeatedly induced to unnatural action to rid the system of this poisonous drug. Nature's efforts are about to cease, and then the patient's suffering life will end."

More deaths have been caused by drug-taking than from all other causes combined. —"How to Live," No. 3, pp. 51–61. Reprinted in *Review and Herald*, Aug. 15–Sept. 12, 1899.

CHAPTER 3

Statements Which May Serve to Define Drugs

Do They Leave Baleful Influences Behind? Nothing should be put into the human system that will leave a baleful influence behind. —*Medical Ministry*, p. 228 (1897).

The simplest remedies may assist nature, and leave no baleful effects after their use. —Letter 82 (1897).

Substances Which Poison the Current of the Blood. In our sanitariums, we advocate the use of simple remedies. We discourage the use of drugs, for they poison the current of the blood. In these institutions sensible instruction should be given how to eat, how to drink, how to dress, and how to live so that the health may be preserved. —*Counsels On Diet And Foods*, p. 303 (1908).

Do not endeavor to adjust the difficulties by adding a burden of poisonous medicines. —*Ministry of Healing*, p. 235 (1905).

Every Pernicious Drug. Every pernicious drug placed in the human stomach, whether by prescription of physicians, or by man himself doing violence to the human organism, injures the whole machinery. — Manuscript 3 (1897).

Break Down Vital Forces. Drugs always have a tendency to break down and destroy vital forces. —*Medical Ministry*, p. 223 (1897).

Poisonous Preparations Which Leave Injurious Effects. God's servants should not administer medicines which they know will leave behind injurious effects upon the system, even if they do relieve present suffering. Every poisonous preparation in the vegetable and mineral kingdoms, taken into the system, will leave its wretched influence, affecting the liver and lungs, and deranging the system generally. —*Spiritual Gifts*, Vol. IV, p. 140 (1864).

Deadly After Effects of Poisonous Drugs. Nature's simple remedies will aid in recovery without leaving the deadly after effects so often felt by those who use poisonous drugs. They destroy the power of the patient to help himself. This power the patients are to be taught to exercise by learning to eat simple, healthful foods, by refusing to overload the stomach with a variety of foods at one meal. All these things should come into the education of the sick. Talks should be given showing how to preserve health, how to shun sickness, how to rest when rest is needed. —Letter 82 (1908) [Physicians and Manager at Loma Linda].

What Are Drugs? [Question to Ellen G. White from a Medical Student.] "Hearing so much about you from my dear mother, knowing how much God has revealed to you concerning this, I have decided to take a little of your time to ask a question which has troubled several of our medical students." Next year a good number of us enter upon our last and most important year of the medical course at the university. From our study of the TESTIMONIES and the little work, HOW TO LIVE, we can see that the Lord is strongly opposed to the use of drugs in our medical work. We believed they were harmful because the Lord had said so through the TESTIMONIES. Now we know from our three years' study that "drugging" is a most unscientific practice.

"Several of the students are in doubt as to the meaning of the word 'drug' as mentioned in HOW TO LIVE. Does it refer only to the stronger medicines as mercury, strychnine, arsenic, and such poisons, the things we medical students call 'drugs,' or does it also include the simpler remedies, as potassium, iodine, squills, etc. We know that our success will be proportionate to our adherence to God's methods. For this reason I have asked the above question." —From Letter Written by Edgar Caro to Mrs. E.G. White, Aug. 15, 1893).

[Ellen G. White's Answer.] Your questions, I will say, are answered largely, if not definitely, in HOW TO LIVE. Drug poisons mean the articles which you have mentioned. The simpler remedies are less harmful in proportion to their simplicity; but in very many cases these are used when not at all necessary. There are simple herbs and roots that every family may use for themselves, and need not call a physician any sooner than they would call a lawyer. I do not think that I can give you any definite line of medicines compounded and dealt out by doctors, that are perfectly harmless. And yet it would not be wisdom to engage in controversy over this subject.

The practitioners are very much in earnest in using their dangerous concoctions, and I am decidedly opposed to resorting to such things. They never cure; they may change the difficulty to create a worse one. Many of those who practice the prescribing of drugs, would not take the same or give them to their children. If they have an intelligent knowledge of the human body, if they understand the delicate, wonderful human machinery, they must know that we are fearfully and wonderfully made, and that not a particle of these strong drugs should be introduced into this human living organism.

As the matter was laid open before me, and the sad burden of the result of drug medication, the light was given me so that Seventh-day Adventists should establish health institutions, discarding all these health-destroying inventions, and physicians should treat the sick upon hygienic principles. The great burden should be to have well-trained nurses, and well-trained medical practitioners to educate "precept upon precept; line upon line, line upon line; here a little, and there a little."

Train the people to correct habits and healthful practices, remembering that an ounce of prevention is of more value than a pound of cure. Lectures and studies in this line will prove of the highest value. — Letter 17-a (1893).

CHAPTER 4

Drugs as Employed in Medical Practice

Poisonous Drugs Which Kill or Leave Baleful Influences Drug medication is to be discarded. On this point the conscience of the physician must ever be kept tender, and true, and clean. The inclination to use poisonous drugs, which kill, if they do not cure, needs to be guarded against. Matters have been laid open before me in reference to the use of drugs. Many have been treated with drugs, and the result has been death. Our physicians, by practicing drug medication, have lost many cases that need not have died if they had left their drugs out of the sick-room.

Fever cases have been lost, when, had the physicians left off entirely their drug treatment, had they put their wits to work, and wisely and persistently used the Lord's own remedies, plenty of air and water, the patients would have recovered. The reckless use of these things that should be discarded has decided the case of the sick.

Experimenting in drugs is a very expensive business. Paralysis of the brain and tongue is often the result, and the victims die an unnatural death, when, if they had been treated perseveringly, with unwearied, unrelaxed diligence with hot and cold water, hot compresses, packs, and dripping sheet, they would be alive today.

Nothing should be put into the human system that will leave a baleful influence behind. And to carry out the light on this subject, to practice hygienic treatment, is the reason which has been given me for establishing sanitariums in various localities.

I have been pained when many students have been encouraged to go where they would receive an education in the use of drugs. The light I have received on the subject of drugs is altogether different from the use made of them at these schools or at the sanitariums. We must become enlightened on these subjects.

The intricate names given medicines are used to cover up the matter, so that none will know what is given them as remedies unless they obtain a dictionary to find out the meaning of these names.

Patients are to be supplied with good, wholesome food; total abstinence from all intoxicating drinks is to be observed; drugs are to be discarded, and rational methods of treatment followed. The patients must not be given alcohol, tea, coffee, or drugs; for these always leave traces of evil behind them. By observing these rules, many who have been given up by the physicians may be restored to health.

In this work the human and divine instrumentalities can cooperate in saving life, and God will add His blessing. Many suffering ones not of our faith will come to our institutions to receive treatment. Those whose health has been ruined by sinful indulgence, and who have been treated by physicians till the drugs administered have no effect, will come; and they will be benefited.

The Lord will bless institutions conducted in accordance with His plans. He will cooperate with every physician who faithfully and conscientiously engages in this work. He will enter the rooms of the sick. He will give wisdom to the nurses. —*Medical Ministry*, pp. 227–229 (Manuscript 162, 1897).

A Terrible Account to Be Rendered to God There is a terrible account to be rendered to God by men who have so little regard for human life as to treat the body so ruthlessly in dealing out their drugs. It is the duty of every person to become intelligent in regard to disease and its causes. We must study our Bible in order to understand the value that the Lord places upon the men and women whom Christ has purchased at such an infinite price. Then we should become acquainted with the laws of life, that every action of the human agent may be in perfect harmony with the laws of God. When there is so great peril in ignorance, is it not best to be wise in regard to the human habitation, fitted up by our Creator, and over which He desires we shall be faithful stewards? We are not excusable if through ignorance we destroy God's building by taking into our stomachs poisonous drugs under a variety of names we do not understand. It is our duty to refuse all such prescriptions. —Manuscript 44 (1896).

Out of Accord With God's Plan. The use of drugs is not in accordance with God's plan. Physicians should understand how to treat the sick through the use of nature's remedies. Pure air, pure water, healthful exercise should be employed in the treatment of the sick...

Many indulge in unhealthful practices until the physical vitality is undermined, and the mental and moral powers are enfeebled. When they fall a prey to disease they resort to drugs, and if these afford them temporary relief, they seem to be satisfied to continue in transgression. They do not bring their habits and practices in review to see what is wrong, and correct the evils by removing the cause. As the drugs are a mere stimulant, after a time they realize that they are in a worse condition than before they used the remedies. To use drugs while continuing evil habits, is certainly inconsistent, and greatly dishonors God by dishonoring the body which He has made. Yet for all this, stimulants and drugs continue to be prescribed, and freely used by human beings, while the hurtful indulgences that produced the disease are not discarded. They use tea, coffee, tobacco, opium, wine, beer, and other stimulants, and give to nature a false support. —Letter 19 (1892) [Dr. Kellogg].

Originated in Perverted Knowledge. From beginning to end, the crime of tobacco using, of opium and drug medication, has its origin in perverted knowledge. It is through plucking and eating of poisonous fruit, through the intricacies of names that the common people do not understand, that thousands and ten thousands of lives are lost. This great knowledge, supposed by men to be so wonderful, God did not mean that man should have. They are using the poisonous productions that Satan himself has planted to take the place of the tree of life, whose leaves are for the healing of the nations. Men are dealing in liquors and narcotics that are destroying the human family. —*Temperance*, p. 75 (Manuscript 119, 1898).

Lack of Faith Made Up by Use of Drugs Those who see Christ by living faith, those who abide in Him, will have power to work miracles for His glory. This is why the physicians and nurses in our medical institutions should be those who abide in Christ; for through their connection with the heavenly Physician their patients will be blessed. These God-fearing workers will have no use for poisonous drugs. They will use the natural agencies that God has given for the restoration of the sick. Time and again I have told the workers in our sanitariums that from the light that God has given me, I know that they need not lose one patient suffering from a fever, if they take the case in hand in time and use rational methods of treatment instead of drugs...

When we are willing to have our own minds unsoldered, and resoldered, by the melting influences of the Spirit of God, we shall understand with new enlightenment Christ's instruction to us as recorded in the fourteenth, fifteenth, sixteenth, and seventeenth chapters of John. O how great are the possibilities that He has placed within our reach! He says, "Whatsoever ye shall ask the Father in my name, he will give it you." He promises to come to us a Comforter to bless us. Why do we not believe these promises? That which we lack in faith we make up by the use of drugs. Let us give up the drugs, believing that Jesus does not desire us to be sick, and that if we live according to the principles of health reform, He will keep us well. —Manuscript 169 (1902) [The Work of the St. Helena Sanitarium].

Easier to Use Drugs. The question is, will they preserve the principles of hygiene, or will they use the easier method of using drugs, to take the place of treating diseases without resorting to drug medication? There could be many hygienic institutions in all parts of our world, if there were plenty of means and plenty of persons who had the qualifications to manage such institutions. —Manuscript 22 (1887).

Not Natural to Laws of Life. Ill health in a variety of forms, if effect could be traced to the cause, would reveal the sure-result of flesh eating. The disuse of meats, with healthful dishes nicely prepared to take the place of flesh meats, would place a large number of the sick and suffering ones in a fair way of recovering their health, without the use of drugs. But if the physician encourages a meat-eating diet to his invalid patients, then he will make a necessity for the use of drug....

Drugs always have a tendency to break down and destroy vital forces, and nature becomes so crippled in her efforts, that the invalid dies, not because he needed to die, but because nature was outraged. If she had been left alone, she should have put forth her highest efforts to save life and health. Nature wants none of such help as so many claim that they have given her. Lift off the burdens placed upon her, after the customs of the fashion of this age, and you will see in many cases nature will right herself. The use of drugs is not favorable or natural to the laws of life and health. The drug medication gives nature two burdens to bear, in the place of one. She has two serious difficulties to overcome, in the place of one. —*Medical Ministry*, pp. 222, 223 (Manuscript 22, 1887).

Drugs and Narcotics Used by Worldly Physicians We should not use the drugs and narcotics used by worldly physicians to relieve the necessity which the abuse of appetite has created in the physical structure. —Letter 56 (1898) [Bro. and Sr. John Wessels].

Use Nature's Remedies. Use nature's remedies—water, sunshine, and fresh air. Do not use drugs. Drugs never heal; they only change the features of the disease. — Letter 116 (1903) [Drs. Kress].

Effects of Pernicious Drugs. Every pernicious drug placed in the human stomach, whether by prescription of physicians or by man himself doing violence to the human organism, injures the whole machinery. Every intemperate indulgence of lustful appetite is at war with natural instinct and the healthful condition of every nerve and muscle and organ of the wonderful human machinery which through the Creator's power possesses organic life.

Nature would do her work wisely and well if the human agent would, in his treatment of the body, cooperate with the divine purpose. But how Satan and his whole confederacy rejoice to see how easily his powers of deception and art can persuade men to form an appetite for most unpleasant stimulants and narcotics. And then when nature has been overborne, enfeebled in all her working force, there is the drug medication to come from the physicians, to kill the remaining vital force and leave men miserable wrecks of suffering, of imbecility, of insanity, and of loathsome disease. God is hidden from the human observation by the hellish shadow of Satan. —Manuscript 3 (1897) [Health Reform].

The Usual Course in the Free Use of Poisonous Drugs A practice that is laying the foundation of a vast amount of disease and of even more serious evils, is the free use of poisonous drugs. When attacked by disease, many will not take the trouble to search out the cause of their illness. Their chief anxiety is to rid themselves of pain and inconvenience. So they resort to patent nostrums, of whose real properties they know little, or they apply to a physician for some remedy to counteract the result of their misdoing, but with no thought of making a change in their unhealthful habits. If immediate benefit is not realized, another medicine is tried, and then another. Thus the evil continues.

People need to be taught that drugs do not cure disease. It is true that they sometimes afford present relief, and the patient appears to recover as the result of their use; this is because nature has sufficient vital force to expel the poison and to correct the conditions that caused the disease. Health is recovered in spite of the drug. But in most cases the drug only changes the form and location of the disease. Often the effect of the poison seems to be overcome for a time, but the results remain in the system and work great harm at some later period.

By the use of poisonous drugs, many bring upon themselves lifelong illness, and many lives are lost that might be saved by the use of natural methods of healing. The poisons contained in many so-called remedies create habits and appetites that mean ruin to both soul and body. Many of the popular nostrums called patent medicines, and even some of the drugs dispensed by physicians, act a part in laying the foundation of the liquor habit, the opium habit, the morphine habit, that are so terrible a curse to society.

The only hope of better things is in the education of the people in right principles. Let physicians teach the people that restorative power is not in drugs, but in nature. Disease is an effort of nature to free the system from conditions that result from a violation of the laws of health. In case of sickness, the cause should be ascertained. Unhealthful conditions should be changed, wrong habits corrected. Then nature is to be assisted in her effort to expel impurities and to reestablish right conditions in the system.

Pure air, sunlight, abstemiousness, rest, exercise, proper diet, the use of water, trust in divine power—these are the true remedies. Every person should have a knowledge of nature's remedial agencies and how to apply them. It is essential both to understand the principles involved in the treatment of the sick and to have a practical training that will enable one rightly to use this knowledge.

The use of natural remedies requires an amount of care and effort that many are not willing to give. Nature's process of healing and upbuilding is gradual, and to the impatient it seems slow. The surrender of hurtful indulgences requires sacrifice. But in the end it will be found that nature, untrammeled, does her work wisely and well. Those who persevere in obedience to her laws will reap the reward in health of body and health of mind. —*Ministry of Healing*, pp. 126, 127 (1905).

Strong, Health-destroying Medicine. Knowledge is what is needed. Drugs are too often promised to restore health, and the poor sick are so thoroughly drugged with quinine, morphine, or some strong health-and-life-destroying [medicine], that nature may never make sufficient protest, but give up the struggle; and they may continue their wrong habits with hopeful impunity. —Manuscript 22 (1887) [To sanitariums].

Interfering with Nature's Laws. Thousands need to be educated patiently, kindly, tenderly, but decidedly, that nine-tenths of their complaints are created by their own course of action. The more they introduce drugs into the system, the more certainly do they interfere with the laws of nature and bring about the very difficulties they drug themselves to avoid. —Manuscript 22 (1887) [To sanitariums].

Weaken the System. Many act as if health and disease were things entirely independent of their conduct, and entirely outside their control. They do not reason from cause to effect, and submit to feebleness and disease as a necessity. Violent attacks of sickness they believe to be special dispensations of Providence, or the result of some overruling, mastering power; and they resort to drugs as a cure for the evil. But the drugs taken to cure the disease weaken the system. —*Medical Ministry*, pp. 296, 297 (Letter 5, 1904).

Drugs Given to Stupefy. Drugs given to stupefy, whatever they may be, derange the nervous system. —*How to Live*, No. 3, p. 57 (1865).

Blood and Bones Poisoned. Brother B seeks to have his wife believe as he believes, and he would have her think that all he does is right and that he knows more than any of the ministers and is wise above all men. I was shown that in his boasted wisdom he is dealing with the bodies of his children as he is with the soul of his wife. He has been following a course according to his own wisdom, which is ruining the health of his child. He flatters himself that the poison which he has introduced into her system keeps her alive. What a mistake! He should reason how much better she might have been had he let her alone and not abused nature. This child can never have a sound constitution, for her bones and the current of blood in her veins have been poisoned. The shattered constitutions of his children and their aches and distressing pains will cry out against his boasted wisdom, which is folly. —*Testimonies*, vol. 3, p. 454 (1875).

Add Not the Burden of Poisonous Medicines. When the abuse of health is carried so far that sickness results, the sufferer can often do for himself what no one else can do for him. The first thing to be done is to ascertain the true character of cause. If the harmonious working of the system has become unbalanced by overwork, overeating, or other irregularities, do not endeavor to adjust the difficulties by adding a burden of poisonous medicines. —*Ministry of Healing*, p. 235 (1905).

Why Some Physicians Prescribe Drugs. The sick are in a hurry to get well, and the friends of the sick are impatient. They will have medicine and if they do not feel that powerful influence upon their systems their erroneous views lead them to think they should feel, they impatiently change for another physician. The change often increases the evil. They go through a course of medicine equally as dangerous as the first. —*How to Live*, No. 3, p. 62 (1865).

Substituting Drugs for Judicious Nursing. There is a disposition with many parents, to keep up a perpetual dosing of their children with medicines. They will always have a supply on hand, and when any slight indisposition is manifested, caused by overeating or exhaustion, the medicine is poured down their throats; and if that does not satisfy them, they send for the doctor. If he is an honest physician, and declines to give the child medicine because he is wise enough to know it will be for its hurt, the parents are offended and think the physician inefficient, and send for another, who is less conscientious, and who will give medicine to satisfy the parents, who were blinded by ignorance in regard to the real condition and need of the child. And not infrequently parents are so anxious to do all they can to save their child, that they change physicians, having two or three to attend the same case. The child is drugged to death, and the parents console themselves that they have done all they could, and wonder why it must die when they did so much to save it. Upon the gravestone of that child should be written, DIED OF DRUG MEDICATION. —"Many Parents Substitute Drugs for Judicious Nursing," *Health Reformer* (Sept. 1886).

Used to counteract Results of Wrongdoing. Men and women use drugs of every description to counteract the results of their own misdoings. Then they charge their suffering to the providence of God, and finish the business by calling in a physician, who drugs to death the remaining forces of nature.

This is a matter of grave responsibility. God holds men and women accountable to keep themselves in the very best health, physically, mentally, and morally, that they may distinguish between the sacred and the common. The laws which God has established for the well-being of the physical structure are to be treated as divine. To every action done in violation of these laws a penalty is affixed. The transgressor is recorded as having broken the commandments of God.

Many seem to think that it is their privilege to treat their bodies as they please. Do such stop to consider that God requires them to obey His physical laws, and that for their violation of these laws they must answer at His bar? —Manuscript 155 (1899) [Temperance from a Christian Standpoint].

Relief Without Drugs. Today Christ is feeling the woes of every sufferer. He would bring relief without the use of drugs. —Manuscript 18 (1898).

Simple Life vs. Drugstore. Thousands who are afflicted might recover their health, if instead of depending upon the drugstore for their life, they would discard all drugs, and live simply, without using tea, coffee, liquor, or spices, which irritate the stomach and leave it weak, unable to digest even simple food without stimulation. The Lord is willing to let His light shine forth in clear, distinct rays to all who are weak and feeble. —*Medical Ministry*, p. 229 (Manuscript 115, 1903).

An Entire Absence of Drugs. A simple diet, and the entire absence of drugs, leaving nature free to recuperate the wasted energies of the body, would make our sanitariums more effectual in restoring the sick to health…

There is need that temperance in eating, drinking, and building be practiced. There is need to educate the people in right habits of living. Put no confidence in drug medicine. If every particle of it were buried in the great ocean, I would say, Amen, for physicians are not working on a right plan. A reform is needed which will go deeper, and be more thorough. —Letter 73-a (1896) [A doctor and his wife].

Abandon Forever. My dear friends, instead of taking a course to baffle disease, you are petting it and yielding to its power. You should avoid the use of drugs and carefully observe the laws of health. If you regard your life you should eat plain food, prepared in the simplest manner, and take more physical exercise. Each member of the family needs the benefits of health reform. But drugging should be forever abandoned; for while it does not cure any malady, it enfeebles the system, making it more susceptible to disease. —*Testimonies,* vol. 5, p. 311 (1889).

CHAPTER 5

Balancing Statements Which May Help Us Find Our Way

Educate Away From — Use Them Less and Less. Among the greatest dangers to our health institutions is the influence of physicians, superintendents, and helpers who profess to believe the present truth, but who have never taken their stand fully upon health reform. Some have no conscientious scruples in regard to their eating, drinking, and dressing. How can the physician or anyone else present the matter as it is when he himself is indulging in the use of harmful things? God's blessing will rest upon every effort made to awaken an interest in health reform, for it is needed everywhere. There must be a revival in regard to this matter; for God purposes to accomplish much through this agency.

Drug medication, as it is generally practiced, is a curse. Educate away from drugs. Use them less and less, and depend more upon hygienic agencies; then nature will respond to God's physicians—pure air, pure water, proper exercise, a clear conscience. Those who persist in the use of tea, coffee, and flesh meats will feel the need of drugs, but many might recover without one grain of medicine if they would obey the laws of health. Drugs need seldom be used. —*Counsels on Health*, p. 261 ("Health and Medical Missionary Work," pp. 42–43; written in 1890).

Seek to Lessen Their Use. In their practice, the physicians should seek more and more to lessen the use of drugs instead of increasing it.... Thus our people, who had been taught to avoid drugs in almost every form, were receiving a different education. —Letter 26a (1889).

Work Away From Drugs. Trust not to your own human wisdom. Trust not in poisonous drugs, that will interfere with nature's work, and leave their cruel trail behind. Work away from drugs, and never, never advise one under your influence to go to Ann Arbor or any place to obtain the education supposed to be essential for the perfection of the medical practitioner. The stamp left upon them by such places is almost ineffaceable. Educate, educate, educate, by placing yourself and others in the closest connection with the greatest Healer the world has ever known. —Letter 40 (1899) [Dr. Kellogg].

Discarding Almost Entirely. Our institutions are established that the sick may be treated by hygienic methods, discarding almost entirely the use of drugs. —*Healthful Living*, p. 246 (1896).

Strong Drugs Need Not Be Used. The first labors of a physician should be to educate the sick and suffering in the very course they should pursue to prevent disease. The greatest good can be done by our trying to enlighten the minds of all we can obtain access to, as to the best course for them to pursue to prevent sickness and suffering, and broken constitutions, and premature death. But those who do not care to undertake work that taxes their physical and mental powers will be ready to prescribe drug medication, which lays a foundation in the human organism for a twofold greater evil than that which they claim to have relieved.

A physician who has the moral courage to imperil his reputation in enlightening the understanding by plain facts, in showing the nature of disease and how to prevent it, and the dangerous practice of resorting to drugs, will have an uphill business, but he will live and let live ... He will, if a reformer, talk plainly in regard to the false appetites and ruinous self-indulgence, in dressing, in eating and drinking, in overtaxing to do a large amount of work in a given time, which has a ruinous influence upon the temper, the physical and mental powers....

Right and correct habits, intelligently and perseveringly practiced, will be removing the cause for disease, and the strong drugs need not be resorted to. Many go on from step to step with their unnatural indulgences, which is bringing in just as unnatural a condition of things as possible. — *Medical Ministry*, pp. 221, 222 (Manuscript 22, 1887).

As It Is Generally Practiced. Drug medication, as it is generally practiced, is a curse. —*Healthful Living*, p. 246.

Less Dangerous if Wisely Administered. Do not administer drugs. True, drugs may not be as dangerous wisely administered as they usually are, but in the hands of many will be hurtful to the Lord's property. — Letter 3 (1884) [Friends at Health Retreat].

Seldom Needed—Use Them Less and Less. Educate people in the laws of life so that they may know how to preserve health. The efforts actually put forth at present are not meeting the mind of God. Drug medication is a curse to this enlightened age.

Educate away from drugs. Use them less and less, and depend more upon hygienic agencies; then nature will respond to God's physicians— pure air, pure water, proper exercise, a clear conscience.

Many might recover without one grain of medicine, if they would live out the laws of health. Drugs need seldom be used. It will require earnest, patient, protracted effort to establish the work and to carry it forward upon hygienic principles. But let fervent prayer and faith be combined with your efforts, and you will succeed. By this work you will be teaching the patients, and others also, how to take care of themselves when sick, without resorting to the use of drugs. —*Medical Ministry*, pp. 259, 260 (Letter 61, 1890).

Discarding Almost Entirely. The use of drugs in our institutions, to the extent to which they are used, is a libel upon the name of hygienic institutions for the treatment of the sick. —Letter 1 (1892) [Brethren Who Stand in Responsible Positions].

Our institutions are established that the sick may be treated by hygienic methods, discarding almost entirely the use of drugs.... There is a terrible account to be rendered to God by men who have so little regard for human life as to treat the body so ruthlessly in dealing out their drugs.... We are not excusable if through ignorance we destroy

God's building by taking into our stomachs poisonous drugs under a variety of names we do not understand. It is our duty to refuse all such prescriptions.

We wish to build a sanitarium [in Australia] where maladies may be cured by nature's own provisions, and where the people may be taught how to treat themselves when sick; where they will learn to eat temperately of wholesome food, and be educated to refuse all narcotics—tea, coffee, fermented wines, and stimulants of all kinds—and to discard the flesh of dead animals. —*Temperance*, pp. 88, 89 (Manuscript 44, 1896).

Finally Cease to Deal Out Drugs. When you understand physiology in its truest sense, your drug bills will be very much smaller, and finally you will cease to deal out drugs at all. The physician who depends upon drug medication in his practice, shows that he does not understand the delicate machinery of the human organism. He is introducing into the system a seed crop that will never lose its destroying properties throughout the lifetime. I tell you this because I dare not withhold it. Christ paid too much for man's redemption to have his body so ruthlessly treated as it has been by drug medication.

Years ago the Lord revealed to me that institutions should be established for treating the sick without drugs. Man is God's property, and the ruin that has been made of the living habitation, the suffering caused by the seeds of death sown in the human system, are an offense to God. —*Medical Ministry*, p. 229 (Letter 73, 1896).

CHAPTER 6:

The Call for the Use of Simple Remedies

The Method Heaven Approves. There are many ways of practicing the healing art, but there is only one way that Heaven approves. God's remedies are the simple agencies of nature that will not tax or debilitate the system through their powerful properties. Pure air and water, cleanliness, a proper diet, purity of life, and a firm trust in God are remedies for the want of which thousands are dying; yet these remedies are going out of date because their skillful use requires work that the people do not appreciate. Fresh air, exercise, pure water, and clean, sweet premises are within the reach of all with but little expense; but drugs are expensive, both in the outlay of means and in the effect produced upon the system.

The work of the Christian physician does not end with healing the maladies of the body; his efforts should extend to the diseases of the mind, to the saving of the soul....

The physician should know how to pray. In many cases he must increase suffering in order to save life; and whether the patient is a Christian or not, he feels greater security if he knows that his physician fears God. Prayer will give the sick an abiding confidence; and many times if their cases are borne to the Great Physician in humble trust, it will do more for them than all the drugs that can be administered. —*Testimonies*, vol. 5, p. 443 (1885).

Use the Simplest Remedies. Nature will want some assistance to bring things to their proper condition, which may be found in the simplest remedies, especially in the use of nature's own furnished remedies —pure air, and with a precious knowledge of how to breathe; pure water, with a knowledge of how to apply it; plenty of sunlight in every room in the house if possible, and with an intelligent knowledge of what advantages are to be gained by its use. All these are powerful in their efficiency, and the patient who has obtained a knowledge of how to eat and dress healthfully, may live for comfort, for peace, for health; and will not be prevailed upon to put to his lips drugs, which, in the place of helping nature, paralyzes her powers. If the sick and suffering will do only as well as they know in regard to living out the principles of health reform perseveringly, then they will in nine cases out of ten recover from their ailments.

The feeble and suffering ones must be educated line upon line, precept upon precept, here a little and there a little, until they will have respect for and live in obedience to the law that God has made to control the human organism. Those who sin against knowledge and light, and resort to the skill of a physician in administering drugs, will be constantly losing their hold on life. The less there is of drug dosing, the more favorable will be their recovery to health. Drugs, in the place of helping nature, are constantly paralyzing her efforts. —*Medical Ministry*, pp. 223, 224 (Manuscript 22, 1887).

Go to the Lord's Dispensary. Christ desires His people to be medical missionaries, able to do His will because they are acquainted with His principles of healing, and are prepared to use the remedies that He Himself has provided in the form of sunshine, pure air, and water. Thousands who go down to the grave might be healed if they would go to the Lord's dispensary rather than to the drugs that man provides. —Letter 30 (1903) [Bro. Murphet].

Combat Disease with Simple Methods. Our people should become intelligent in the treatment of sickness without the aid of poisonous drugs. Many should seek to obtain the education that will enable them to combat disease in its varied forms by the most simple methods. Thousands have gone down to the grave because of the use of poisonous drugs, who might have been restored to health by simple methods of treatment. Water treatments, wisely and skillfully given, may be the means of saving many lives. —*Medical Ministry*, p. 227 (Manuscript 15, 1911).

To Restore Health, But Not With Drugs. Physicians are placed in positions of temptation and danger. But they may stand firm to their allegiance if they will take hold of the strength that God offers them. He says, "Let him take hold of my strength, that he may make peace with me, and he shall make peace with me." The Lord will be the helper of every physician who will work together with Him in the effort to restore suffering humanity to health, not with drugs, but with nature's remedies. Christ is the great Physician, the wonderful Healer. He gives success to those who work in partnership with Him. —Letter 142 (1902) [Bro. W.H. Jones].

Drugs Not Sanctioned by Christ. In the Saviour's manner of healing, there were lessons for His disciples. On one occasion He anointed the eyes of a blind man with clay, and bade him, "Go, wash in the pool of Siloam … He went his way therefore, and washed, and came seeing" [John 9:7]. The cure could be wrought only by the power of the great Healer, yet Christ made use of the simple agencies of nature. While He did not give countenance to drug medication, He sanctioned the use of simple and natural remedies.…

We should teach others how to preserve and to recover health. For the sick we should use the remedies which God has provided in nature, and we should point them to Him who alone can restore. —*Desire of Ages*, p. 824 (1898).

Water vs. Poisonous Drugs. It is not safe to trust to physicians who have not the fear of God before them. Without the influence of divine grace the hearts of men are "deceitful above all things, and desperately wicked." Self-aggrandizement is their aim. Under the cover of the medical profession what iniquities have been concealed, what delusions supported!...

Go with me to yonder sickroom. There lies a husband and father, a man who is a blessing to society and to the cause of God. He has been suddenly stricken down by disease. The fire of fever seems consuming him. He longs for pure water to moisten the parched lips, to quench the raging thirst, and cool the fevered brow. But, no, the doctor has forbidden water. The stimulus of strong drink is given and adds fuel to the fire. The blessed, heaven-sent water, skillfully applied, would quench the devouring flame; but it is set aside for poisonous drugs.

For a time nature wrestles for her rights; but at last, overcome, she gives up the contest, and death sets the sufferer free. God desired that man to live, to be a blessing to the world; Satan determined to destroy him, and through the agency of the physician he succeeded. How long shall we permit our most precious lights to be thus extinguished? —*Testimonies*, vol. 5, pp. 194, 195 (1882).

Water Treatments Given Skillfully. Our sanitariums should be established in retired places, that are free from all noise and confusion, such as the rumbling of carriages and streetcars.

The Lord has taught us that great efficacy for healing lies in a proper use of water. These treatments should be given skillfully. We have been instructed that in our treatment of the sick we should discard the use of drugs. There are simple herbs that can be used for the recovery of the sick, whose effect upon the system is very different from that of those drugs that poison the blood and endanger life. —Manuscript 73 (1908) [Counsels Repeated].

Natural Surroundings and Hydrotherapy More Effective Than Drugs. The things of nature are God's blessings, provided to give health to body, mind, and soul. They are given to the well to keep them well and to the sick to make them well. Connected with water treatment, they are more effective in restoring health than all the drug medication in the world. —*Testimonies*, vol. 7, p. 76 (1902).

A Lesson From Hezekiah's Experience. The Lord will heal those who believe, but He has given natural blessings for the benefit of the afflicted, and He would have these used. God could have healed Hezekiah with a word. But He heard Hezekiah's prayer, and gave directions that a bunch of figs be placed upon the diseased parts. This was done, and Hezekiah recovered. But his recovery was not instantaneous. He had not the same faith that the afflicted woman had. We need to exercise faith. To practice the use of drug medication does not harmonize with faith. Appealing to worldly physicians is dishonoring to God. Those who come to God in faith must cooperate with Him in accepting and using His heaven-sent remedies—water, sunlight, and plenty of air.

It is of no use to have seasons of prayer for the sick, while they refuse to use the simple remedies which God has provided, and which are close by them. If there is an unsanitary condition of things in the house and about the premises, the very first thing is to take up the work that has been neglected, and cleanse and purify the house and premises, making everything sweet, that the atmosphere may not be tainted by the least offensive smell. —Letter, 106 (1898) [Bro. Chapman].

Simple Preparations vs. Drug Medication. The drug science has been exalted, but if every bottle that comes from every such institution were done away with, there would be fewer invalids in the world today. Drug medication should never have been introduced into our institutions. There was no need of this being so, and for this very reason the Lord would have us establish an institution (in Australia) where He can come in and where His grace and power can be revealed. "I am the Resurrection and the Life," He declares.

The true method for healing the sick is to tell them of the herbs that grow for the benefit of man. Scientists have attached large names to these simplest preparations, but true education will lead us to teach the sick that they need not call in a doctor any more than they would call in a lawyer. They can themselves administer the simple herbs if necessary. To educate the human family that the doctor alone knows all the ills of infants and persons of every age is false teaching, and the sooner we as a people stand on the principles of health reform, the greater will be the blessing that will come to those who would do true medical work. There is a work to be done in treating the sick with water, and teaching them to make the most of the sunshine and physical exercise. Thus in simple language we may teach the people how to preserve health, how to avoid sickness. This is the work our sanitariums are called upon to do. This is true science. — Manuscript 105 (1898) [The Education Our School Should Give].

Antidotes for Disease in Simple Plants. Christ never planted the seeds of death in the system. Satan planted these seeds when he tempted Adam to eat of the tree of knowledge, which meant disobedience to God. Not one noxious plant was placed in the Lord's great garden, but after Adam and Eve sinned, poisonous herbs sprang up. In the parable of the sower the question was asked the Master, "Didst not thou sow good seed in thy field? How then hath it tares?" The Master answered, "An enemy hath done this." All tares are sown by the evil one. Every noxious herb is of his sowing, and by his ingenious methods of amalgamation he has corrupted the earth with tares.

Then shall physicians continue to resort to drugs which leave a deadly evil in the system, destroying that life which Christ came to restore? Christ's remedies cleanse the system. But Satan has tempted man to introduce into the system that which weakens the human machinery, clogging and destroying the fine, beautiful arrangements of God. The drugs administered to the sick do not restore, but destroy. Drugs never cure. Instead, they place in the system seeds which bear a very bitter harvest....

Our Saviour is the restorer of the moral image of God in man. He has supplied in the natural world remedies for the ills of man, that His followers may have life and that they may have it more abundantly. We can with safety discard the concoctions which man has used in the past. The Lord has provided antidotes for disease in simple plants, and these can be used by faith, with no denial of faith; for by using the blessings provided by God for our benefit we are cooperating with Him. He can use water and sunshine and the herbs which He has caused to grow in healing maladies brought on by indiscretion or accident. We do not manifest a lack of faith when we ask God to bless His remedies. True faith will thank God for the knowledge of how to use these precious blessings in a way which will restore mental and physical vigor. —Manuscript 65 (1899).

Value of Roots and Herbs. If we neglect to do that which is within the reach of nearly every family, and ask the Lord to relieve pain, when we are too indolent to make use of these remedies within our power, it is simply presumption. The Lord expects us to work in order that we may obtain food. He does not propose we shall gather the harvest unless we break the sod, till the soil, and cultivate the produce. Then God sends the rain and the sunshine and the clouds to cause vegetation to flourish. God works and man cooperates with God. Then there is seedtime and harvest. God has caused to grow out of the ground herbs for the use of man, and if we understand the nature of these roots and herbs, and make a right use of them, there would not be a necessity of running for the doctor so frequently, and people would be in much better health than they are today. —*Medical Ministry*, pp. 230, 231 (Letter 35, 1890).

Other Simple Remedies. The intricate names given the medicines are used to cover up the matter, so that none will know what is given them as remedies unless they obtain a dictionary to find out the meaning of these names. The Lord has given some simple herbs of the field that at times are beneficial; and if every family were educated in how to use these herbs in case of sickness, much suffering might be prevented, and no doctor need be called. These old-fashioned, simple herbs, used intelligently, would have recovered many sick, who have died under drug medication.

One of the most beneficial remedies is pulverized charcoal, placed in a bag and used in fomentations. This is a most successful remedy. If wet and in smartweed boiled, it is still better. I have ordered this in cases where the sick were suffering great pain, and when it has been confided to me by the physician that he thought it was the last before the close of life. Then I suggested the charcoal, and the patient slept, the turning point came, and recovery was the result. To students when injured with bruised hands and suffering with inflammation, I have prescribed this simple remedy, with perfect success. The poison of inflammation was overcome, the pain removed, and healing went on rapidly. The most severe inflammation of the eyes will be relieved by a poultice of charcoal, put in a bag, and dipped in hot or cold water, as will best suit the case. This works like a charm.

I expect you will laugh at this; but if I could give this remedy some outlandish name, that no one knew but myself, it would have greater influence. But Dr. Kellogg, many things have been opened before me that no one but myself is any the wiser for in regard to the management of sickness and disease—the effect of the use of drug medication, the thousands in our work who might have lived if they had not sent for a physician, and had let nature work the recovery herself. But the simplest remedies may assist nature, and leave no baleful effects after their use. — Letter 82 (1897) [Dr. J. H. Kellogg].

Those Who Make a Practice of Taking Drugs. Your letter to me, under date Feb. 12, is received. Your question is, "Is it advisable to employ a good, Christian physician, who treats his patients on hygienic principles? In urgent cases, should we call in a worldly physician, because the sanitarium doctors are all so busy that they have no time to devote to outside practice? Some say that when the sanitarium doctors do use drugs, they give larger doses than ordinary doctors."

If the physicians are so busy that they cannot treat the sick outside of the institution, would it not be wiser for all to educate themselves in the use of simple remedies, than to venture to use drugs, that are given a long name to hide their real qualities. Why need anyone be ignorant of God's remedies—hot water fomentations and cold and hot compresses. It is important to become familiar with the benefit of dieting in case of sickness. All should understand what to do themselves. They may call upon someone who understands nursing, but everyone should have an intelligent knowledge of the house he lives in. All should understand what to do in case of sickness....

Those who make a practice of taking drugs sin against their intelligence and endanger their whole after-life. There are herbs that are harmless, the use of which will tide over many apparently serious difficulties. But if all would seek to become intelligent in regard to their bodily necessities, sickness would be rare instead of common. An ounce of prevention is worth a pound of cure. —Manuscript 86 (1897) [Health Reform Principles].

Medicinal Properties of the Trees. In a certain place, preparations were being made to clear the land for the erection of a sanitarium. Light was given that there is health in the fragrance of the pine, the cedar, and the fir. And there are several other kinds of trees that have medicinal properties that are health-promoting. Let not such trees be ruthlessly cut down. Better change the site of the building than cut down these evergreen trees. —Letter 95 (1902) [Brethren Kilgore and Jacobs].

Better Than Drugs. I have been unable to sleep after half-past eleven at night. Many things, in figures and symbols, are passing before me. There are sanitariums in running order near Los Angeles. At one place there is an occupied building, and there are fruit trees on the sanitarium grounds. In this institution, outside the city, there is much activity.

As in the vision of the night I saw the grounds, I said, "O ye of little faith! You have lost time." There were sick in wheelchairs. There were some patients to whom the physicians had given a prescription to spend all their time outdoors during pleasant weather, in order to regain health....

While speaking, I said: "We must have sanitariums in favored places in different localities. This is God's plan. He has ordained the medical missionary work as a means of saving souls, and that which we see about us is a symbol of the work before us. We are to awaken our churches to engage interestedly in God's work, and to carry forward this branch—the medical missionary work."

Physicians were interested in these words, and one said, as he extended his arms and waved them back and forth, "Is not this better than drugs? Aches and pains have left you without the use of medicine."

On the grounds that I saw in this vision of the night, there were shade trees, the boughs of which were hung in such a way that they formed leafy canopies somewhat the shape of tents. The sick were delighted. While some were working for diversion, others were singing. There was no dissatisfaction. —Manuscript 152 (1901) [Brethren and Sisters in Southern California].

Exercise Better Than Medicine. Inactivity is the greatest curse that could come upon most invalids. Light employment in useful labor, while it does not tax mind and body, has a happy influence upon both. It strengthens the muscles, improves the circulation, and gives the invalid the satisfaction of knowing that he is not wholly useless in this busy world. He may be able to do but little at first, but he will soon find his strength increasing and the amount of work done can be increased accordingly. Exercise aids the dyspeptic by giving the digestive organs a healthy tone....

Those whose habits are sedentary should, when the weather will permit, exercise in the open air every day, summer or winter. Walking is preferable to riding or driving, for it brings more of the muscles into exercise. The lungs are forced into healthy action, since it is impossible to walk briskly without inflating them. Such exercise would in many cases be better for the health than medicine. —*Ministry of Healing*, p. 240 (1905).

Bring Into Prominence Healing Without Drugs. In every large city there should be a representation of true medical missionary work. Let many now ask: "Lord, what wilt Thou have me to do?" (Acts 9:6). It is the Lord's purpose that His method of healing without drugs shall be brought into prominence in every large city through our medical institutions. God invests with holy dignity those who go forth farther and still farther, in every place to which it is possible to obtain entrance. —*Testimonies*, vol. 9, p. 169 (1905).

Use Intelligently God's Restoring Agencies. The ambassadors of Christ can be doubly useful if they know how to restore the diseased to health. This was the work of Christ. But as in prayer we present these suffering ones to the Lord for His healing power to come to them, the people themselves must be instructed to do those things which will assist nature, not in drug medication, but in the use of the agencies the Lord has prepared—sunlight, pure air, pure water, healthful exercise. These things possess a power which millions in our world know nothing of. These restoring agencies must be used intelligently, and as we do all that it is in our power to do, we must mingle with our work our earnest prayers. — Manuscript 110 (1898).

Simple Methods vs. Poisonous Drugs. Thousands need and would gladly receive instruction concerning the simple methods of treating the sick—methods that are taking the place of the use of poisonous drugs. There is great need of instruction in regard to dietetic reform. Wrong habits of eating and the use of unhealthful food are in no small degree responsible for the intemperance and crime and wretchedness that curse the world. —*Ministry of Healing*, p. 146 (1905).

CHAPTER 7

Medication in Our Sanitariums

Sanitariums to Treat Without Drugs. Our sanitariums are one of the most successful means of reaching all classes of people. Christ is no longer in this world in person, to go through our cities and towns and villages healing the sick. He has commissioned us to carry forward the medical missionary work that He began; and in this work we are to do our very best. Institutions for the care of the sick are to be established, where men and women may be placed under the care of God-fearing medical missionaries and be treated without drugs. To these institutions will come those who have brought disease on themselves by improper habits of eating and drinking. These are to be taught the principles of healthful living. They are to be taught the value of self-denial and self-restraint. They are to be provided with a simple, wholesome, palatable diet and are to be cared for by wise physicians and nurses.

Our sanitariums are the right hand of the gospel, opening doors whereby suffering humanity may be reached with the glad tidings of healing through Christ. In these institutions the sick may be taught to commit their cases to the Great Physician, who will co-operate with their earnest efforts to regain health, bringing to them healing of soul as well as healing of body. —*Counsels on Health*, p. 212 (Review and Herald, March 23, 1905).

Discard in Our Sanitariums. The light given me was that a sanitarium should be established, and that in it drug medication should be discarded, and simple, rational methods of treatment employed for the healing of disease. In this institution people were to be taught how to dress, breathe, and eat properly—how to prevent sickness by proper habits of living. — *Counsels on Diet and Foods*, p. 303 (1905).

Simple Remedies vs. Drugs. It would have been better if, from the first, all drugs had been kept out of our sanitariums, and use had been made of such simple remedies as are found in pure water, pure air, sunlight, and some of the simple herbs growing in the field. These would be just as efficacious as the drugs used under mysterious names, and concocted by human science, and they would leave no injurious effects in the system.

Thousands who are afflicted might recover their health if, instead of depending upon the drug store for their life, they would discard all drugs, and live simply, without using tea, coffee, liquor, or spices, which irritate the stomach, and leave it weak, unable to digest even simple food without stimulation. The Lord is willing to let His light shine forth in clear, distinct rays to all who are weak and feeble.

Vegetables, fruits, and grains should compose our diet. Not an ounce of flesh-meat should enter our stomachs. The eating of flesh is unnatural. We are to return to God's original purpose in the creation of man. — Manuscript 115 (1903) [Instruction Regarding Sanitarium Work].

Established To Do Away With Drugs. Lead them [the people] away from drug medication, educating them and training them that drugs kill more than they cure. This matter is presented to me so frequently, that I cannot hold my peace upon this subject. The use of poisonous drugs is coming more and more into practice among our people. The light which the Lord has given me is, that institutions should be established to do away with drugs, and use God's agencies; that instruction should be given daily upon this subject. But God's ways and instruction have not been heeded, therefore not one-twentieth part of the good has been accomplished which might have been if Christian physicians had heeded the admonitions and the counsel of the Most High. —Letter 21c (1892) [Dr. and Mrs. Maxson].

When the Sanitarium Was First Established. As matters have been opened to me from time to time, as I have been conducted through the rooms of the sick in the Sanitarium and out of the Sanitarium, I have seen that the physicians of the Sanitarium, by practicing drug medication, have lost many cases that need not have died if they had left their drugs out of the sick room. Cases have been lost that, had the physicians left off entirely their drug treatment, had they put their wits to work, and wisely and persistently used the Lord's own remedies, plenty of air and water—the fever cases that have been lost would have recovered. The reckless use of those things that should be discarded has decided the case of the sick.

I will not educate or sustain the use of drugs … After seeing so much harm done by the administering of drugs, I cannot use them, and cannot testify in their favor. I must be true to the light given me by the Lord.

The treatment we gave when the Sanitarium was first established required earnest labor to combat disease. We did not use drug concoctions; we followed hygienic methods. This work was blessed by God. It was a work in which the human instrumentality could cooperate with God in saving life. There should be nothing put into the human system that would leave its baleful influence behind. And to carry out the light on this subject, to practice hygienic treatment, and to educate on altogether different lines of treating the sick, was the reason given me why we should have sanitariums established in various localities. I have been pained when many students have been encouraged to go Ann Arbor, to receive an education in the use of drugs. The light which I have received has placed an altogether different complexion on the use made of drugs than is given at Ann Arbor or at the Sanitarium. We must become enlightened on these subjects. — Letter 82 (18970 [To Dr. Kellogg].

Sanitariums Without Drug Medication. The light was given that we should have a sanitarium, a health institution, which was to be established right among us. This was the means God was to use in bringing His people to a right understanding in regard to health reform. It was also to be the means by which we were to gain access to those not of our faith. We were to have an institution where the sick could be relieved of suffering, and that without drug medication. God declared that He Himself would go before His people in this work. —Manuscript 150 (1901) [Give the Medical Missionary Work Its Place].

Educate Patients Away From Drugs. We are health reformers. Physicians should have wisdom and experience, and be thorough health reformers. Then they will be constantly educating by precept and example their patients from drugs. For they well know that the use of drugs may produce for the time being favorable results, but will implant in the system that which will cause great difficulties hereafter, which they may never recover from during their lifetime. Nature must have a chance to do her work. —*Medical Ministry*, pp. 224, 225 (Manuscript 22, 1887).

Our sanitariums are established as institutions where patients and helpers may serve God. We desire to encourage as many as possible to act their part individually in living healthfully. We desire to encourage the sick to discard the use of drugs, and to substitute the simple remedies provided by God, as they are found in water, in pure air, in exercise, and in general hygiene. —Manuscript 115 (1907) [Why We Have Sanitariums, an Address at Dedicatory Services of the St. Helena Sanitarium].

Lessen Use of Drugs. In their practice, the physicians should seek more and more to lessen the use of drugs instead of increasing it. When Dr. — came to the Health Retreat, she laid aside her knowledge and practice of hygiene, and administered the little homeopathic doses for almost every ailment. This was against the light God had given. Thus our people, who had been taught to avoid drugs in almost every form, were receiving a different education. I was obliged to tell her that this practice of depending upon medicine, whether in large or small doses, was not in accordance with the principles of health reform. The Lord had in His providence given light in regard to the establishment of sanitariums where the sick should be treated upon hygienic principles. The people must be taught to depend on the Lord's remedies, pure air, pure water, simple, healthful foods....

Physicians have a work to do to bring about reform by educating the people, that they may understand the laws which govern their physical life. They should know how to eat properly, to work intelligently, and to dress healthfully, and should be taught to bring all their habits into harmony with the laws of life and health, and to discard drugs. There is a great work to be done. If the principles of health reform are carried out, the work will indeed be as closely allied to that of the third angel's message as the hand is to the body....

If they move in God's way, physicians of the same faith will be linked together in a strong brotherhood, aiding one another to reach the highest standard, and devise means to enlighten the people, not encouraging in the use of drugs, but leading away from drug medication. Teach the people how to prevent disease. Tell them to cease rebelling against nature's laws, and by removing every obstruction, give her a chance to put forth her very best efforts to set things right. Nature must have a fair chance to employ her healing agencies. We must make earnest efforts to reach a high platform in regard to the methods of treating the sick. If the light which God has given prevails, if truth overcomes error, advanced steps will be taken in health reform. This must be. —Letter 26a (1889) [Dr. and Mrs. Maxson].

Work Away From as Fast as Possible. The Health Retreat [St. Helena Sanitarium] was established at a great cost to treat the sick without drugs. It should be conducted on hygienic principles. Drug medication should be worked away from as fast as possible, until entirely discarded. Education should be given on proper diet, dress, and exercise. Not only should our own people be educated, but those who have not received the light upon health reform should be taught how to live healthfully, according to God's order. —Letter 3 (1884).

Sanitariums Using Simple Remedies. Small sanitariums are to be connected with our schools. The students are to be taught how to use nature's simple remedies in the treatment of disease. And as they learn to care for the sick, they are to be taught to act under the direction of the Lord Jesus Christ. —*Review and Herald* (Sept. 9, 1902).

Institutions Treating Without Drugs. The question of health reform is not agitated as it must and will be. A simple diet, and the entire absence of drugs, leaving nature free to recuperate the wasted energies of the body, would make our sanitariums far more effectual in restoring the sick to health. —*Temperance*, p. 89 (Letter 73a, 1896).

Institutions for the care of the sick are to be established, where men and women suffering from disease may be placed under the care of God-fearing physicians and nurses, and be treated without drugs. —Letter 305 (1905) [Mr. Walter Harper].

One patient, successfully treated, will have a testimony to bear of the virtue of the simple methods of treatment, the simple, healthful remedies that nature has provided, without the use of any drugs. —Letter 53 (1905) [Brethren Ballenger and Palmer].

CHAPTER 8

Ellen G. White and Her Use of Remedies

The Use of Remedies to Alleviate Pain. It is not a denial of faith to use such remedies as God has provided to alleviate pain and to aid nature in her work of restoration … We should employ every facility for the restoration of health, taking every advantage possible, working in harmony with natural laws. —*Ministry of Healing*, pp. 231, 232 (1905).

It is no denial of faith to use rational remedies judiciously. Water, air, and sunshine, these are God's healing agencies. The use of certain herbs that the Lord has made to grow for the good of man, is in harmony with the exercise of faith. —Manuscript 31 (1911).

Determined to Know the Medicine She Took. Were I sick, I would just as soon call in a lawyer as a physician from among general practitioners. I would not touch their nostrums, to which they give Latin names. I am determined to know, in straight English, the name of everything that I introduced into my system. —Manuscript 86 (1897) [Health Reform Principles].

E.G. White Refused Drugs. Last night I spent many wakeful hours in prayer. I am resolved to cast myself, body, soul, and spirit, upon the Lord. I cannot take drugs. They do me no good, but harm. I long for the blessing of the Lord. My heart goes out after God. I tremble at His word.

I am encouraged as I look to Jesus and recount His loving-kindnesses: "In my distress I called upon the Lord, and cried unto my God; He heard my voice out of His temple, and my cry came before Him, even into His ears." "He brought me forth also into a large place; He delivered me, because He delighted in me." "I love the Lord, because He hath heard my voice and my supplications." This has been my experience day and night during my sickness. —Manuscript 20 (1892) [Diary written in Preston, Victoria, Australia, relating to her ten months of suffering from rheumatic fever].

Combating Inflammation with Charcoal. On one occasion a physician came to me in great distress. He had been called to attend a young woman who was dangerously ill. She had contracted fever while on the campgrounds and was taken to our school building, near Melbourne, Australia. But she became so much worse that it was feared she could not live. The physician, Dr. Merritt Kellogg, came to me and said, "Sister White, have you any light for me on this case? If relief cannot be given our sister, she can live but a few hours." I replied, "Send to a blacksmith's shop and get some pulverized charcoal; make a poultice of it, and lay it over her stomach and sides." The doctor hastened away to follow out my instructions. Soon he returned, saying, "Relief came in less than half an hour after the application of the poultices. She is now having the first natural sleep she has had for days."

I have ordered the same treatment for others who were suffering great pain, and it has brought relief, and been the means of saving life. My mother had told me that snake bites and the sting of reptiles and poisonous insects could often be rendered harmless by the use of charcoal poultices. When working on the land at Avondale, Australia, the workmen would often bruise their hands and limbs, and this in many cases resulted in such severe inflammation that the worker would have to leave his work for some time. One came to me one day in this condition, with his hand tied in a sling. He was much troubled over the circumstances; for his help was needed in clearing the land. I said to him, "Go to the place where you have been burning the timber, and get me some charcoal from the eucalyptus tree, and pulverize it, and I will dress your hand." This was done, and the next morning he reported that the pain was gone. Soon he was ready to return to his work.

I write these things that you may know that the Lord has not left us without the use of simple remedies which when used will not leave the system in the weakened condition in which the use of drugs so often leaves it. We need well-trained nurses who can understand how to use the simple remedies that nature provides for restoration to health, and who can teach those who are ignorant of the laws of health how to use these simple but effective cures. —Letter 90 (1908).

Charcoal and Olive Oil. I will tell you a little about my experience which charcoal as a remedy. For some forms of indigestion, it is more efficacious than drugs. A little olive oil into which some of this powder has been stirred tends to cleanse and heal. I find it is excellent…

Always study and teach the use of the simplest remedies, and the special blessing of the Lord may be expected to follow the use of these means which are within the reach of the common people. —Letter 100 (1903).

Eucalyptus and Honey. I have already told you the remedy I use when suffering from difficulties with my throat. I take a glass of boiled honey, and into this I put a few drops of eucalyptus oil, stirring it in well. When the cough comes on, I take a teaspoonful of this mixture, and relief comes almost immediately. I have always used this with the best results. I ask you to use the same remedy when you are troubled with the cough. This prescription may seem so simple that you feel no confidence in it, but I have tried it for a number of years, and can highly recommend it. —Letter 20 (1909).

I have had considerable trouble with my throat, but whenever I use this [eucalyptus and honey], I overcome the difficulty very quickly. I have to use it only a few times, and the cough is removed. If you will use this prescription, you may be your own physician. If the first trial does not effect a cure, try it again. The best time to take it is before retiring. — Letter 348 (1908).

Leaves from the Eucalyptus Tree. Take warm footbaths, into which have been put the leaves from the eucalyptus tree. There is great virtue in these leaves, and if you will try this, you will prove my words to be true. The oil of the eucalyptus is especially beneficial in case of cough and pains in the chest and lungs. I want you to make a trial of this remedy which is so simple, and which costs you nothing. —Letter 20 (1909).

Red Clover Tea. I have always used red clover tea, as I stated to you. I offered you this, and told you it was a good, simple, and wholesome drink. —Letter 12 (1888).

Simple Herbs. The Lord has given some simple herbs of the field that at times are beneficial; and if every family understood how to use these herbs in case of sickness, much suffering might be prevented, and no doctor need be called. These old-fashioned, simple herbs, used intelligently, would have recovered many sick who have died under drug medication. —Manuscript 162 (1897).

There are herbs that are harmless, the use of which will tide over many apparently serious difficulties. But if all would seek to become intelligent in regard to their bodily necessities, sickness would be rare instead of common. An ounce of prevention is worth a pound of cure. —Manuscript 86 (1897).

A Few Other Simple Remedies. Water can be used in many ways to relieve suffering. Draughts of clear, hot water taken before eating (half a quart, more or less), will never do any harm, but will rather be productive of good. A cup of tea made from catnip herb will quiet the nerves.

Hop tea will induce sleep. Hop poultices over the stomach will relieve pain. If eyes are weak, if there is pain in the eyes, or inflammation, soft flannel cloths wet in hot water and salt, will bring relief quickly.

When the head is congested, if the feet and limbs are put in a bath with a little mustard, relief will be obtained.

There are many more simple remedies, which will do much to restore healthful action to the body. All these simple preparations the Lord expects us to use for ourselves; but man's extremities are God's opportunities.

If we neglect to do that which is within the reach of nearly every family, and ask the Lord to relieve pain, when we are too indolent to make use of these remedies within our power, it is simply presumption. —Letter 35 (1890).

Grape Juice and Eggs. I have told you what I have because I have received light that you are injuring your body by a poverty-stricken diet … It is the lack of suitable food that has caused you to suffer so keenly. You have not taken the food essential to nourish your frail physical strength. You must not deny yourself of good, wholesome food.… Get eggs of healthy fowls. Use these eggs cooked or raw. Drop them uncooked into the best unfermented wine you can find. This will supply that which is necessary to your system. —*Counsels on Diet and Foods*, pp. 203, 204 (1901) [Dr. Kress].

Blood Transfusions. There is one thing that has saved life—an infusion of blood from one person to another; but this would be difficult and perhaps impossible for you to do. I merely suggest it. —Letter 37 (1901) [Dr. Kress].

E. G. White Requests Powders for Cancer Sufferers.

Dr. Gibbs: Dear Brother, I have just received a letter from Brother Stephen Belden of Norfolk Island. He is afflicted with a cancer. Brother Alfred Nobbs, the elder of the Norfolk Island Church, has also been afflicted with what appeared to be a cancer. He went to Sydney, and his face and head were badly cut in removing the cancer. But he received little help, and he still continues to suffer greatly.

Brother Stephen Belden has a cancer on his ear. I thought that if you would send him powders at once, with directions for their use, Brother Belden and Brother Nobbs might both be benefited by their use.

Will you kindly respond by sending the powders as soon as you receive this letter? I am not well today, so cannot write much. I will send you this line, hoping that you will send the powders. —Letter 236 (1906).

Note: The value of this communication lies, not in the powder Dr. Gibbs might suggest which might bring relief in the cancer case, but in the fact that Mrs. White was eager to have use made of a powder she hoped might be a remedy. —A. L. White

Vaccination for Smallpox. [Statement made by D. E. Robinson]. "Though fully aware of the practice of vaccination during an epidemic of smallpox she expressed no disapproval of it either as a preventative or a remedy. Members of her own family were vaccinated with her approval." —*Story of Our Health Message*, appendix (March 1954).

X-Ray Treatments at Loma Linda. For several weeks I took treatment with the x-ray for the black spot that was on my forehead. In all I took twenty-three treatments, and these succeeded in entirely removing the mark. For this I am very grateful. —Letter 30 (1911).

CHAPTER 9

The Several Schools of Medicine

Not to Advocate One Above Another. Physicians should be ambassadors for Christ in their specific work, and instead of giving prominence to a special theory of medicine which they advocate, by a godly life and conversation they should make prominent the fact that they are Christians. Not one of the schools of medicine highly lauded in the world is approved in the courts above, nor do they bear the heavenly superscription and endorsement. You are not justified in advocating one school above the others, as though it were the only one worthy of respect. Those who vindicate one school of medicine and bitterly condemn another are actuated by a zeal that is not according to knowledge.

With what pharisaic pride some men look down upon others who have not received a diploma from the so-called standard school. All this proves that they cannot see afar off, and have not been purged from their old sins. They need to humble themselves at the cross of Calvary. This spirit will never be acknowledged in heaven, nor will men who cherish it hear the "Well done." Some have been as zealous in exalting what their particular school advocated as though the Lord had specified that that method was the only one to be allowed.

The use of drugs has resulted in far more harm than good; and should our physicians who claim to believe the truth almost entirely dispense with medicine, and faithfully practice alone the lines of the principles of hygiene, using nature's remedies, far greater success would attend their efforts. The duties and qualifications of a physician are not small. — *Special Testimonies*, Book D, pp. 270, 271.

As the Talk of the Pharisees. Feeling existed in regard to the method that was used at the Retreat under Dr. A's directions. Dr. A, with the utmost confidence and assurance, extolled the Regular practice, and depreciated the practice of Homeopathy, and made the most extravagant statements in regard to the Regular practice. Some might take these statements as verity and truth, but I knew that they were not correct; for the practice of both systems and their results had been laid open before me, and I knew that the statements that he made were not correct. But this is due to the narrow cut of the mind of the man. The system in which he has been educated he regards as the best of all methods. The Lord regards all this talk just as He regards the talk of the Pharisees—as the invention and tradition of men.

All those who receive their education from the Regular school, and are molded by the spirit of the educators, generally act out the impressions they have received from their instructors, and denounce every other system as Satanic. Is this the way of the Lord? If the priests and Pharisees kept the way of the Lord, then Dr. A's ideas are correct. The use of drugs in our institutions, to the extent to which they are used, is a libel upon the name of hygienic institutions for the treatment of the sick. The physicians need to be converted on this point as decidedly as the sinner needs the converting power of God on life and character in order to become a pure-hearted Christian. Let the students who go to obtain a medical education at the Medical Institute of our land, learn all that they possibly can of the principles of life, but let them discard error, and not become bigots, I would not speak thus plainly, unless I felt that it was necessary. —Letter 1 (1892) [Brethren Who Stand in Responsible Positions].

There Must Be a Reform. In regard to hygienic methods and the misuse of drugs, from the light God has given me, there must be a reform. Our people are going far from the light which God has given on this subject. If Dr. B or Dr. A or any other doctor goes into the institution, he must work in harmony with the light God has seen fit to give to His people in reform methods of treatment. If Dr. and his wife unite with Dr. B or any other physician, all egotism must be done away. The spirit that controlled the medical fraternity has been of that character which will exclude many from heaven unless they put away this spirit and work with the mind and spirit of Christ. Wicked jealousies, evil thinking, evil speaking of their brethren, has been an offence to God. The methods of drug medication have created the bitterest animosity in feeling, almost equal to the prejudice that Catholics have manifested toward Protestants because they did not view every point of religious faith as they themselves.

Such a spirit may be expected in the world, but when it becomes a controlling power among Christians, it is an offence to God. It is a shame when manifested among those who profess to be followers of Jesus. There must be a reform among the medical fraternity or the church will be purged from those who will not be Bible Christians. It is altogether too late in the day for such a Satanic exhibition of spirit as is revealed among medical drug practitioners. God abhors it. I could write much on this subject, but I am not able now. —Letter 48 (1892) [Elder Haskell].

The Spirit of Free Masonry Manifested. I wish I could see you face to face, but as I cannot, I will write. Thank you for your prescription. I will be careful. The Lord help me, is my prayer, and I pray that the Lord may help you, my brother, that you may not take on too many burdens, and by so doing disqualify yourself for the management of them…

The influence you have gained in the medical profession is large and broad, and in some respects it has been as God would have it. You have caused the light God has given you to shine forth to others, and this light has influenced others to labor in the different lines in the medical work. But according to the light the Lord has given me, something of the spirit of Free Masonry exists, and has built a wall about the work. The old regular practice has been exalted as the only true method for the treatment of disease. And to a large degree this feeling has leavened the physicians connected with you. They have resorted to drugs in cases of fever to break it up, as they have thought. This method has broken up fevers and other diseases, but it has in some cases broken up the whole man with it.

The Lord has been pleased to present this matter before me in clear lines. Fever cases need not be treated with drugs. The most difficult cases are best and most successfully managed by nature's own resources. This science, fully adopted, will bring the best results, if the practitioner will be thorough. The Lord will bless the physician who depends on natural methods, helping every function of the human machinery to act in its own strength the part the Lord designed it to act in restoring itself to proper action.

Dr. Kellogg, God has given you favor with the medical fraternity, and He would have you hold that favor. But in no case are you to stand as do the physicians of the world to exalt Allopathy above every other practice, and call all other methods quackery and error; for from the beginning to the present time the results of Allopathy have made a most objectionable showing. There has been loss of life in your sanitarium because drugs have been administered, and these give no chance for nature to do her work of restoration. Drug medication has broken up the power of the human machinery, and the patients have died. Others have carried the drugs away with them, making less effective the simple remedies nature uses to restore the system. The students in your institution are not to be educated to regard drugs as a necessity. They are to be educated to leave drugs alone.

The medical fraternity, represented to me as Free Masonry, with their long, unintelligible names, which common people cannot understand, would call the Lord's prescription for Hezekiah quackery. Death was pronounced upon the king, but he prayed for life, and his prayer was heard. Those who had the care of him were told to get a bunch of figs and put them on the sore, and the king was restored. This means was taken by God to teach them that all their preparations were only depriving the king of the power to rally and overcome disease. While they pursued their course of treatment, his life could not be saved. The Lord diverted their minds from their wonderful mysteries to a simple remedy of nature. There are lessons for us all in these directions. Young men who are sent to Ann Arbor to obtain an education which they think will exalt them as supreme in their treatment of disease by drugs, will find that it will result in the loss of life rather than restoration to health and strength. These mixtures place a double taxation upon nature, and in the effort to throw off the poisons they contain, thousands of persons lose their lives. We must leave drugs entirely alone, for in using them we introduce an enemy into the system. I write this because we have to meet this drug medication in the physicians in this country, and we do not want this practice as in Battle Creek to steal into our midst as a thief. We want the door closed against the enemy before the lives of human beings are imperilled. —Letter 67 (1899) [Dr. Kellogg].

CHAPTER 10

How Our Physicians Should Be Trained

Physicians to Unlearn Much. It would have been better if those sent from our schools to Ann Arbor had never had any connection with that institution. The education in drug medication and the false religious theories have brought forth a class of practitioners who need to unlearn much they have learned. They need to obtain an altogether different experience before they can say in word and in deed, We are medical missionaries. Till they obtain such an experience, the great Physician does not acknowledge them as medical missionaries. They come on to the platform of action unprepared for the high and holy work which needs to be done at this time. —Letter 3 (1901) [Dr. E. R. Caro].

Many Will Never Receive Heavenly Diploma. There is to be a sanitarium in Australia, and altogether new methods of treating the sick are to be practiced. Drug medication must be left out of the question, if the human physician would receive the diploma written and issued in heaven. There are many physicians who will never receive this diploma unless they learn in the school of the great Physician. This means that they must unlearn and cast away the supposed wonderful knowledge of how to treat disease with poisonous drugs. They must go to God's great laboratory of nature, and there learn the simplest methods of using the remedies which the Lord has furnished. When drugs are thrown aside, when fermented liquor of all kinds is discarded, when God's remedies, sunshine, pure air, water, and good food are used, there will be far fewer deaths and a far greater number of cures. —Manuscript 65 (1899).

Loma Linda Students to Learn to Treat Disease Without Poisonous Drugs. The students at Loma Linda are seeking for an education that is after the Lord's order, an education that will help them to develop into successful teachers and laborers for others. When their education at Loma Linda is completed, they should be able to go forth and join the intelligent workers in the world's great harvest fields who are carrying forward the work of reform that is to prepare a people to stand in the day of Christ's coming. Everywhere workers are needed to know how to combat disease and give skillful care to the sick and suffering. We should do all in our power to enable those who desire to be thus fitted for service to gain the necessary training....

Our people should become intelligent in the treatment of sickness without the aid of poisonous drugs. Many should seek to obtain the education that will enable them to combat disease in its various forms by the most simple methods. Thousands have gone down to the grave because of the use of poisonous drugs, who might have been restored to health by simple methods of treatment. Water treatments, wisely and skillfully given, may be the means of saving many lives. Let diligent study be united with careful treatments. Let prayers of faith be offered by the bedside of the sick. Let the sick be encouraged to claim the promises of God for themselves. —*Medical Ministry*, pp. 56, 57 (Manuscript 15, 1911).

Poisonous Drugs Need Not Be Used. Let the students be given a practical education. The less dependent you are upon worldly methods of education, the better it will be for the students. Special instruction should be given in the art of training the sick without the use of poisonous drugs and in harmony with the light that God has given. In the treatment of the sick, poisonous drugs need not be used. Students should come forth from the school without having sacrificed the principles of health reform or their love for God and righteousness.

The education that meets the world's standard is to be less and less valued by those who are seeking for efficiency in carrying the medical missionary work in connection with the work of the third angel's message. They are to be educated from the standpoint of conscience, and, as they conscientiously and faithfully follow right methods in their treatment of the sick, these methods will come to be recognized and preferable to the methods to which many have become accustomed, which demand the use of poisonous drugs.

We should not at this time seek to compete with worldly medical schools. Should we do this, our chances of success would be small. — *Testimonies*, vol. 9, pp. 175, 176 (1909).

Teach Science of Healing Without Drugs. The Lord calls for the best talents to be united at this center [Loma Linda] for the carrying on of the work as He has directed—not the talent that will demand the largest salary, but the talent that will place itself on the side of Christ to work in His lines. We must have medical instructors who will teach the science of healing without the use of drugs.… We are to prepare a company of workers who will follow Christ's methods. —*Medical Ministry*, p. 75 (Letter 196, 1908).

Character of Drugs Concealed by Difficult Names. Let the instruction be given in simple words. We have no need to use the many expressions used by worldly physicians which are so difficult to understand that they must be interpreted by the physician. These long names are often used to conceal the character of the drugs being used to combat disease. We do not need these.

Nature's simple remedies will aid in recovery without leaving the deadly after-effects so often felt by those who use poisonous drugs. — Letter 82 (1908) [Physicians and Manager at Loma Linda].

To Correct False Habits and Practices. The work of the physician must begin in an understanding of the works and teachings of the Great Physician. Christ left the courts of heaven that He might minister to the sick and suffering of earth. We must cooperate with the Chief of Physicians, walking in all humility of mind before Him. Then the Lord will bless our earnest efforts to relieve suffering humanity. It is not by the use of poisonous drugs that this will be done, but by the use of simple remedies. We should seek to correct false habits and practices, and teach the lessons of self-denial. The indulgence of appetite is the greatest evil with which we have to contend. —*Medical Ministry*, p. 85 (Letter 140, 1909).

Not to Be Taught the Use of Drugs. I found an article that I had written about a year ago, in reference to the establishment of a school of the highest order, in which the students would not be taught to use drugs in the treatment of the sick. —Letter 360 (1907).

Competent Physicians to Teach Drugless Therapy. Those who desire to become missionaries are to hear instruction from competent physicians, who will teach them how to care for the sick without the use of drugs. Such lessons will be of the highest value to those who go out to labor in foreign countries. And the simple remedies used will save many lives. —*Medical Ministry*, p. 231 (Manuscript 83, 1908).

Our Physicians Need Not Administer Drugs. It is not necessary that our medical missionaries follow the precise track marked out by medical men of the world. They do not need to administer drugs to the sick. They do not need to follow the drug medication in order to have influence in their work. The message was given me that if they would consecrate themselves to the Lord, if they would seek to obtain under men ordained of God a thorough knowledge of their work, the Lord would make them skillful.

Some of our medical missionaries have supposed that a medical training according to the plans of worldly schools is essential to their success. To those who have thought that the only way to success is by being taught by worldly men and by pursuing a course that is sanctioned by worldly men, I would now say, Put away such ideas. This is a mistake that should be corrected. It is a dangerous thing to catch the spirit of the world; the popularity which such a course invites, will bring into the work a spirit which the Word of God cannot sanction.

It is a lack of faith in the power of God that leads our physicians to lean so much on the arm of the law, and to trust so much to the influence of worldly powers. The true medical missionary will be wise in the treatment of the sick, using the remedies that nature provides. And then he will look to Christ as the true healer of diseases. The principles of health reform brought into the life of the patient, the use of nature's remedies, and the cooperation of divine agencies in behalf of the suffering, will bring success.

I am instructed to say that in our educational work there is to be no compromise in order to meet the world's standards. God's commandment-keeping people are not to unite with the world to carry various lines of work according to worldly plans and worldly wisdom....

Facilities should be provided at Loma Linda, that the necessary instruction in medical lines may be given by instructors who fear the Lord, and who are in harmony with His plans for the treatment of the sick. — *Review and Herald* (March 6, 1913).

CHAPTER 11

Seventh-day Adventists to Influence Medical Practice

To Reform Medical Practices. As to drugs being used in our institutions, it is contrary to the light which the Lord has been pleased to give. The drugging business has done more harm to our world and killed more than it has helped or cured. The light was first given to me why institutions should be established, that is, sanitariums were to reform the medical practices of physicians. —*Medical Ministry*, p 27 (Letter 89, 1898).

What Dr. Kellogg Accomplished. The Lord has connected Dr. Kellogg with the medical fraternity outside our people. His influence has had much to do with the abolishing of drugs to a large extent, and the introduction of nature's own restoratives. This work has not been done by making a raid upon drugs, for it needed the wisdom of a serpent and the harmlessness of a dove. Dr. Kellogg's connection with God enables him to take the presence of the Holy Spirit with him into assemblies where there is generally much levity, and where many things are spoken that might better be left unsaid. The people respect the doctor's religious principles, and show that they are somewhat under the influence of this faith. —Letter 38 (1899) [Elders Prescott, Irwin, Jones, Smith, and Waggoner].

Appendix A

A Letter by Dr. Paulson on the Use of Drugs

(Hinsdale, IL, July 19, 1914)

Dr. Thyra H. Jasselyn (Madison, IN)

Dear Doctor:

A few weeks ago Bro. L. A. Hansen, of the Medical Missionary Department, forwarded to me the following questions which you had raised:

"I cannot understand what Mrs. White means when she says that drugs are not necessary in the treatment of disease unless it is just what she says; but I am told by another Adventist doctor on our staff that I misunderstood her attitude.

"Though I too think that we should not use drugs needlessly, I should not wish to disregard the value of antitoxin in diphtheria, quinine in malaria, etc.

"Other Adventist physicians use such remedies and do not feel that they are in the wrong. I do not see how they reconcile their position with such statements as I enclose."

Brother Hansen suggested my writing something on this question. It is with some hesitancy that I do so, because I feel that on a question of such vital importance if any man speak let him speak as the oracles of God (1

Pet.4:11), and unless God by His grace shall enable me to do that, I feel silence would be golden on my part.

We are naturally inclined to interpret the Testimonies in the light of our own practice instead of humbly acknowledging that we have come short of the glory of God. It is God's plan that the prophets should hew us up to the divine standard (Hos. 6:5), while the tendency of our natural inclinations is to hew the prophets down to the level of our practice. On this question of drug therapy I am quite convinced that the reformers need to be reformed; that in brokenness of heart, like Daniel of old, we need to confess not only the sins of our medical brethren, but our own individual sins as well.

Some twenty odd years ago a group of us medical students left the Battle Creek Sanitarium and went to Ann Arbor to begin our medical course. Some of us made a most careful and prayerful study from the Bible and Testimonies of fundamental medical missionary principles including, of course, therapeutics. We soon became convinced that there were some remedies that God has promised to especially bless, that there were others to which He could not in a similar signal manner add His blessing.

Dr. Oslar, now of Oxford, England, but then of John Hopkins, had just issued his first edition of his famous textbook on the practice of medicine. It was the most radical departure from the old therapeutic program that had ever appeared, and he speedily and justly earned the title of a therapeutic annihilist as far as drugs were concerned. It was evident to any careful observer that Dr. Oslar paced little or no reliance in drug therapy. This naturally made it easier for some of us to take the various statements in the Testimonies more nearly at their par value.

Some of our number naturally undertook to harmonize the statements with their particular modified beliefs on the questions. This led Bro. Caro, my roommate, to write to Sister White some questions very similar to the ones you have raised. I am enclosing you a copy of her entire reply as far as it had any bearing whatsoever on this subject. Summed up in a nutshell, there is no repudiation of the former statements made; rather, the enunciation of this self-evident principle, that the simpler remedies are less harmful in proportion to their simplicity; that there are "herbs and roots" that every family may use for themselves as opposed to "dangerous concoctions." In a later unpublished testimony, written Aug. 26, 1895, I quote the following:

"Many of the physicians in our world are of no benefit to the human family. The drug science has been exalted, but if every bottle that comes from every such institution were done away with, there would be fewer invalids in the world today. Drug medication should never have been introduced into our institutions. There was no need of this being so, and for this reason the Lord would have established an institution where He can come in and where His grace and power can be revealed, 'I am the resurrection and the life,' He declares.

"The true method of healing the sick is to tell them of the herbs that grow for the benefit of man. Scientists have attached large names to these simplest preparations, but true education will lead us to teach the sick that they need not call in a doctor any more than they would call in a lawyer. They themselves administer the simple herbs if necessary. To educate the human family that the doctor alone knows all the ills of infants and persons of every age is false teaching, and the sooner we as a people stand on the principles of health reform, the greater will be the blessing that will come to those who would do true medical missionary work. There is a work to be done in treating the sick with water, teaching them to make the most of the sunshine and physical exercise. Thus in simple language we may teach the people how to preserve health, how to avoid sickness. This is the work our sanitariums are called upon to do. This is true science." —E. G. White, Manuscript 105 (1898).

Here is a clean-cut statement that drug medication should never have been introduced into our institutions. At the same time, the point is emphasized that there are herbs that grow for the benefit of man. The administering of these "simple herbs if necessary" is put alongside the standing "on the principles of health reform" and "treating the sick with water" and "sunshine and physical exercise."

It is evident even after all this instruction has been imparted to us on the subject of drug medication, that there is still, as always is the case, a twilight zone where the human agent must use his own sanctified judgment in making the full application. The Lord never deals with us in arbitrary terms. He still leaves plenty of necessity of seeing Him for individual light.

It is very evident that, humanly speaking, it would be much more desirable if the Testimonies should have specifically pointed out senna, for instance, as a simple herb that might properly be used, while on the other hand, nux vomica, as the Testimonies have already stated, is a drug that never should be used.

But, as I have stated above, much of the Lord's instructions is in general principles sufficiently plain that those who earnestly desire to do His will at any cost may, by the aid of the Holy Spirit, learn to apply it, while those who want to follow their own inclinations will have abundant excuse for doing so.

Instead of finishing at the University of Michigan, I graduated at Bellevue Medical College, New York City. The learned professor of medicine enthusiastically recommended alcohol as the important remedy in various infectious diseases. Knowing that the Bible had declared it to be a deceiver, and that the Testimonies have unqualifiedly condemned it, all this false instruction did not influence me a hair's breadth. Naturally it is gratifying to me to have lived long enough to find no intelligent up-to-date physician today who believes alcohol is anything but a detriment in the sick room.

When we became physicians in the Battle Creek Sanitarium some of us earnestly insisted that such drugs as strychnine, calomel, and others that had been specifically pointed out as always injurious to the human system should be repudiated by the institution. I am glad to say that Dr. Kellogg took the same position, said that he never had any faith in them, that they had been dragged into the institution by some of the practitioners who had been taught in medical schools that they were valuable remedies.

Naturally the argument that morphine was justifiable and essential to subdue the pain after an operation as was chloroform during an operation seemed unanswerable, and perhaps is et in some instances unanswerable. However, I remember more than one case where even at the midnight hour some of us gathered in some quiet room and unitedly presented some poor sufferer's case to God in prayer, and were gratified to find ere we had finished our prayer the patient had dropped off into a sweet refreshing sleep, from which he awoke entirely free from pain.

Mind you, none of us took the position that morphine should never be used; we simply insisted, knowing its dangerous character, having abundant opportunity to see the poor drug slaves as they were drifting in there to be cured of its awful tyranny, that morphine should not be injected into a patient until God's remedies, prayerfully applied, had had fair opportunity to demonstrate what was God's will in that particular case.

Naturally quinine was considered just as indispensable in malaria as morphine was following certain surgical operations. We soon had an abundant opportunity to put our principles in regard to quinine to a practical test. It happened to be a malarial summer in Michigan. During the summer something like fifty cases came to us in all ages and in all stages of the disease. Dr. Kress and I, who could not consistently reconcile the prevailing routine quinine program with some of the truths we had studied, determined we would discover for ourselves what God would help us to do in malarial cases without quinine. One member of our class was an enthusiastic advocate of quinine. It was mutually agreed that as the patients came in, one was to be assigned to this physician, the next one to be assigned to Dr. Kress and myself, and so alternating. As he was also a microscopic expert, having taken special training in blood work, every case, not only his but ours, was carefully checked up by himself by laboratory work, so there was no chance for guesswork. It was probably as fair a test as was ever made.

We carefully took the temperature every fifteen minutes. As soon as there began to be the least rise of temperature that was a notification to us that the chill was approaching, we at once put the patient into a hot blanket pack, which brought on profound perspiration, and thereby if we had it right we would invariably prevent the chill. The patients would perspire for a time, we would take them out carefully, provided it was the alternate day variety we gave them tonic treatments. The following day we again instituted the temperature-taking program. We invariably found that the rise of temperature was much delayed, showing that we were gaining the ascendancy. We would then go through the same program. Frequently we did not have to do this the third time; the work had been done, and in a week or ten days the patient was fully restored to health. Sometimes we would miss hitting it just right for several days, so there would be a delay.

Now for comparison: the quinine certainly enabled the malarial patients to recover; but it was the after-history where the tremendous difference was shown. Not one of our cases had serious complications. One of them (of the other group) has gone through life since practically deaf. Another one had his mentality greatly impaired, so far as I know it has remained so to this day. Still others had minor complications.

One day an old, feeble, broken-down man came in so loaded with malaria that it seemed as though he was on the brink of the grave. According to the rotation he belonged on the quinine list. The doctor, after sizing up the situation, said he did not dare to undertake his case, so he was turned over to our list. I will never forget when Dr. Kress and I went over to the Cushman Cottage and earnestly told the Lord that His principles were on test, and pleaded with Him to vindicate what He had said. We then took hold of the case. Within a week the man was restored to health.

Metchnikoff, head of the Pasteur Institute, in his book *The New Hygiene*, says: "It is not only opium and alcohol which hinder the phagocytic action. A number of other substances regularly employed in medicine cause the same results. Even quinine, the prophylactic effect of which in malarial fevers is indisputable, is a poison for the white blood cells. One should, therefore, as a general rule avoid as far as possible the use of all sorts of medicaments, and limit oneself to the hygienic measures which may check the outbreak of infectious diseases. This postulate further strengthens the thesis that the future of medicine rests far more in hygiene than in therapeutics."

The remarkable work that has been done the last few years in the Tulane University, New Orleans, by one of the professors who has succeeded for the first time in cultivating malarial parasites in test tubes, outside the body, shows plainly why we are able to succeed without packs. And he is already raising the question whether our old notion of how the quinine killed the parasites is not erroneous; in other words, the quinine probably only enables the body to handle the parasites just as the packs do, only in a much more expensive way to the body. If that is so, then of course that becomes one more striking commentary on that statement in the Testimonies, that the use of drugs by our practitioners is merely a confession of the ignorance of physiology and how to use nature's remedies successfully.

Shortly after I took charge of the nervous department of the Battle Creek Sanitarium a prominent businessman came up from Chicago. He was suffering with progressive atrophy of the left shoulder and upper arm, the muscles having already largely shrunk away. His case had been diagnosed by one of Chicago's leading neurologists who, having had his attention called to the fact that Dr. Gower in England had reported some apparent improvement in sever cases by the use of strychnine injections, recommended that he should have strychnine injections in connection with sanitarium treatments.

I knew that the Testimonies had declared that strychnine had no business in the human body, and my conscience simply would not permit this as long as the man was under my care, even though an eminent physician in Chicago had ordered it to be done. I was compelled to explain to the man my conscientious scruples in regard to this; told him that if he insisted on having this strychnine injection he would have to go back to his Chicago doctor. He naturally said to me, "Will you promise to cure me with your sanitarium remedies without strychnine?" I told him no, progressive atrophy was considered an incurable disorder by any methods. He said he could not see the consistency of my position when the nerve specialist in Chicago had held out some hopes from strychnine when I did not dare to hold out positive hope with physiological measures. I told him that I was more anxious to be right than he was to be consistent, and that I was managing my department for God, that I had conscientious scruples against the use of strychnine and hence simply would not use it, but if he wanted to have it used it was proper to avail himself of the same; but in order to do so he would have to seek it elsewhere. He remarked that he did not know anything about my God, but did know he wanted to get well. But instead of going away he remained. In six weeks' time his muscles were fully filled in. A few years ago I dropped into the Battle Creek Sanitarium, and this man happened to be back there. He came up and introduced himself and called my attention to the fact that his shoulder was all right up to date.

I draw no lessons from this; I am simply stating my experience. But this thing I do know that every time we compromise we may miss a providence. And furthermore, those who compromise what they know to be principle are always in the fog, and in a little while their conscience becomes as clastic as India rubber, and it seems to be their lot and misfortune to be constantly brought into apparently impossible situations where they cannot, as far as they can see, possibly get out without further compromising principles; while God neve permits the man of unswerving principle to get into a situation where he considers he has any good excuse for compromising even as much as a hair's breadth what he knows to be right.

Priessnitz, as you well know, established and maintained in Silicia, Austria, years ago a successful absolutely drugless institution. The royalty of Europe were among his patrons. Eminent men whose cases had baffled the skill of our best physicians went even from our own land to that out-of-the-way place, and were restored to health by his drugless methods. It was not a fad that lasted merely a year or two, but it went on year after year until it became the most notable center in the world. Cures were constantly being accomplished that seemed nothing short of miraculous. I have naturally been interested in that work, and I have in my library today something like twenty different books bearing on Priessnitz' work. Some of them were written by eminent physicians who themselves went there either to investigate the merits of the institution or as patients. All without exception bore testimony to the marvelous cures that this man Priessnitz secured by using nature's remedies exclusively.

The day may not be far distant when the Lord will raise up some Seventh-day Adventist Priessnitz who will effectually put to silence the lingering doubts, the apparently unsurmountable objections to carrying out literally the program outlined for us in the Testimonies. In fact, the prevailing medical practice is many days' journey nearer that ideal today than it was in Priessnitz' time. I attended the meeting of the American Medical Association a year ago in Minneapolis. My wife, Dr. Mary Paulson, attended different sections than I did so we might between us gather as many helpful facts as possible. She said that she didn't hear during the time we were there a single drug recommended by any speaker. Dr. Cabot of Harvard was the only man who recommended a single drug remedy in my hearing, and that was large doses of bismuth for dysentery; but he knew that it could do no harm. The entire emphasis was laid upon the very remedies that the Testimonies have pointed out over and over again during these fifty years.

You raise the question of the use of antitoxin in diphtheria, to which I would briefly say that until I get more light than I have now, I consider it just as natural to go to the horse for antitoxin if the child is short on its own account, as it is to go to the cow for milk when the child's mother is short in this respect.

I said in the beginning of this letter that it is with much hesitancy that I write you what I am doing, for it is with a deep sense of my own short-comings in this respect. However, that you may know that this whole matter is still a matter of conscience with me, I shall enclose a copy of some correspondence that I have had just recently with a prominent physician who sent me a case of pernicious anemia with beginning of a serious nerve complication. When the doctor ordered hypodermic injections of arsenate of iron, I tried to soothe my conscience with the fact that it was his responsibility and not mine; that if I refrained from doing it the patient would get the same treatment at home anyway, and he would miss the sanitarium treatments which he so much needed. But I speedily discovered that I could not make this reasoning square with my conscience, and I had to go through the humiliating experience of writing what I did, which was probably no easier for me to do than it would have been for you or anyone else under similar circumstances. It is not a particularly pleasant performance to go down in the dust, although I know from previous experience that it brings the peaceful fruits of righteousness to those who are exercised thereby.

Last year we had a case of pernicious anemia here whose life hung on a thread; hemoglobin 20, red blood cells much less than a million. I had telegraphed her husband to be here, as she was about to pass away. At this juncture she whispered in Mrs. Paulson's ear, "Pray." She sent for me. We knelt down together at the woman's bedside. She was a devout woman, though not a Seventh-day Adventist. We prayed the Lord if it pleased Him to restore this woman to health. From that day she began to improve rapidly, and in three months' time she went home a well woman. More than a year has passed by, and she is still, at the latest reports I have had, as well as ever.

I have seen such things happen to often to juggle with my conscience so God should be compelled to rob me of these experiences. It is when we are in a crisis, it is when we do not know what to do next, if we endeavor to take one more step, then it is that God invariably meets us. He does not always restore our sick to health, but He gives us the signal satisfaction that we are His servants, that we have done all things at His word (1 Kings 18:36).

In Vol. 9, page 175, are found these significant words:

Special instruction should be given in the art of treating the sick without the use of POISONOUS drugs, and in harmony with the light that God has given ... They are to be educated from the standpoint of CONSCIENCE, and as they conscientiously and faithfully follow right methods in their treatment of the sick, these methods will come to be recognized as PREFERABLE to the methods to which many have become accustomed, which demand the use of poisonous drugs. [Emphasis mine]

How can we possibly do that unless we are willing to pay the price of having a clear-cut conscience of our own? Our nurses need to be taught that God has promised to link His blessing with the remedies that He Himself has designated rather than with those that He has condemned.

"There are many ways of practicing the healing art, but there is only one way that heaven approves. God's remedies are the simple agencies of nature, that will not tax or debilitate the system through their powerful properties" (vol. 5, p. 443).

I fear that I have not satisfactorily answered your question. I feel humble under a sense of my own short-comings; but I feel determined to continue to press toward the light to spell out more and more faithfully God's program.

[Signed] Yours in the Master's Work,

David Paulson, M. D.

Appendix B

Questions

The following are questions that if prayerfully considered will help one answer the questions about the application of this counsel to the present day, and whether the use of modern drugs is an acceptable form of treatment for the sick in the eyes of God.

1) The Lord has told us which healing agencies He approves the use of—pure air, pure water, sunlight, abstemiousness, rest, exercise, proper diet, cleanliness, trust in divine power. Were these remedies adequate back then? Are they adequate today?

2) If drugs were to change and become beneficial where they were once harmful, why did our Lord not foresee the change and tell us about it? If the counsel concerning drugs was very soon to become obsolete, why was so much counsel given on the subject?

3) How is it possible to determine the effect of drugs when many of the effects are delayed for years and manifest themselves in the form of unrelated diseases?

4) The present line of medicine that is now declared to be beneficial and reasonably safe would not have been invented if we had followed God's counsel. Can something good for the human race come through disobedience to God?

5) Can S. D. A. medical practice today—which is virtually identical to what the world has to offer—be considered the right arm and entering

wedge of a message that is to be distinct and far above what the world has to offer?

6) When we consider God's healing agencies are only effective when used by those who believe in the efficiency, and are obedient to God's methods of healing, then can a physician who was trained for years in the use of drugs be objective on the subject of God's healing agencies, when he was never trained in their use or observed their effect?

7) If research proved the Lord's counsel to be true concerning medicine would we then discard the use of these things? If so who are we putting our faith in? If we wait until then, how are we to be the head and not the tail? How are we to reform medical practice unless we believe the counsel on drugs now?

8) Do our physicians who believe in drugs also advocate and rely largely on the use of God's healing agencies? Do they educate their patients concerning all the laws of health and urge them to be obedient to these laws?

9) Who gets the credit for healing when drugs are used? If our doctors were really giving credit to God, why do they insist on using drugs that God condemns in the first place? How much honor do we give to God when we say that for Him to heal someone He needs the help of our man-made drugs?

10) Is it possible that medical schools that were educating in the use of harmful drugs in Ellen White's day, started educating in the use of safe drugs shortly after her death? At what point were medical schools converted to the ways that God approves?

11) Since it is only the power of Christ that heals disease, by what power do Godless physicians appear to heal disease? Can true healing take place apart from Christ? Does Christ give His power to those who reject His love and His law?

12) If God's chosen method today is the use of drugs, then why are so many diseases on the increase? Why are there any sick among us?

13) Where did we get our present knowledge of drugs from? Did we get it from God or did we seek it from those who are disobedient to the commandments of God, those whose education we were to value less and less?

14) Since we are promised the restoration of, and the maintaining of health if we trust in God and faithfully obey His health laws, where do drugs fit into that kind of a program?

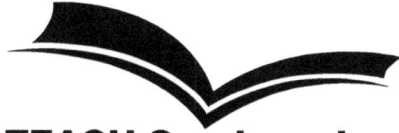